THE UNOFFICIAL GUIDE TO PRACTICAL SKILLS

FIRST EDITION

Emily Hotton
Zeshan Qureshi

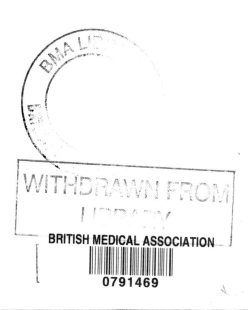

ISBN 978-0957149960
Text, design and illustration © Zeshan Qureshi 2014

Edited by Emily Hotton and Zeshan Qureshi

Published by Zeshan Qureshi. First published 2014

Original design by Zeshan Qureshi and Emily Hotton. Front cover design by Zeshan Qureshi, Emily Hotton, and Tom Green. Page make-up by Anchorprint Group Limited

Illustrated by Anchorprint Group Limited, Peter Gardiner: medical illustrations (clinical skills limited) and Martin Burnett: clinical photographs (UK Media Solutions)

A catalogue record for this book is available from the British Library.

Publisher and Chief Editors' Acknowledgements:
We would like to thank all the authors for their hard work, and our distinguished panel of expert reviewers for their specialist input. We are extremely grateful for the support given by medical schools across the UK. We would also like to thank the medical students that have inspired this project, believed in this project, and have helped contribute to, promote, and distribute the book across the UK.

Thank you to Matt Harris, Andrew Strain, Baldeep Sidhu, Kyle Gibson, and Reza Jarral for their contributions to the Practical Skills chapter of the Unofficial Guide to Passing OSCEs upon which this book has been developed.

Thank you to Ruth Harrison, Srikant Ganesh, Abiola Adeogun for acting as models. Particular thanks go to Natalie Blencowe, for her constant advice and support. We also want to make a special mention to Dr and Mrs Hotton, who have been truly invaluable in providing energy and support to see this project through. Thanks also go to the Bath Academy, at the University of Bristol for the equipment and facilities for the images.

The authors and publishers would like to thank the following for permission to reproduce their images:
Reproduced by the kind permission of the Resuscitation Council (UK): Fig 3.7, 3.10, 3.13
Dr David Pothier (www.earatlas.co.uk): 3.70, 3.71, 3.72, 3.73, 3.74, 3.75
Pamela Gulland/Hannah Collinson: ECG 1-6 (Station 3.9)
Dr Richard Mansfield: Fig 3.56, 3.60, 3.61
Dr Ed Friedlander: Fig 3.66
NHS Lothian: Fig 3.65, 3.68
NHS Fife: Fig 3.64, 3.67
CME Medical UK Ltd: Fig 4.16

Commissioned photographs by:
Katrina Mason: All images: station 5.13
Martin Burnett (www.martinburnettphotography.co.uk): All other photographs

Commissioned medical illustrations by:
Peter Gardiner (petergardiner@clinicalskills.net)

Printed and bound by Cambrian Printers in UK

INTRODUCTION

'The Unofficial Guide to Practical Skills' follows on from the huge success of 'The Unofficial Guide to Passing OSCEs'. This book covers the core clinical competencies for new graduates, as well as additional practical procedures that are expected to be performed by junior doctors. Written by recently qualified foundation doctors, with review by senior clinicians, we have ensured that all procedures follow current guidelines.

This book has detailed explanations of over 50 practical skills stations. Each station includes a corresponding mark scheme, associated questions and answers as well as further areas to explore. The aim is to give you a comprehensive overview of all procedures, even if you have yet to witness them in your training. Covering both basic and more advanced practical skills, we hope this book will prove to be a handy study companion for your undergraduate and postgraduate training.

Practical procedures can be nerve-wracking to perform, both under the close scrutiny of OSCE examiners and pressures of daily clinical practice. The following simple measures are central to performing practical skills proficiently and effectively:

... take time to prepare yourself for the procedure

... ensure you are familiar with the method and equipment you need

... make sure that correct infection control measures are undertaken, from hand washing to use of personal protective items

... always identify the patient you are about to perform a procedure on and obtain the appropriate consent

... check the patient understands your explanation and allow time for them to ask any questions

... be confident in your ability

... use the experience of your peers

... if you are having difficulty, seek help

With this textbook, we hope you will become more confident and competent in these skills both in exams and in clinical practice, but we hope that this is just the beginning. We want you to get involved, this textbook has been written by junior doctors and students just like you because we believe:

... that fresh graduates have a **unique perspective** on what works **for students.** We have tried to capture the insight of students and recent graduates to make the language we use to discuss this complex material more digestible **for students.**

... that texts are in **constant** need of being updated. **Every student** has the potential to contribute to the education of others by innovative ways of thinking and learning. This book is an open collaboration with you.

You have the power to **contribute** something valuable to medicine; we welcome your suggestions and would love for you to get in touch. A good starting point is our facebook page, which is growing into a forum for medical education, search for "The Unofficial Guide to Medicine" or enter the hyperlink below into your web browser.

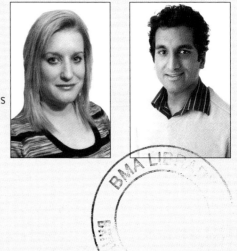

Please get in touch and be part of the medical education project

Emily: emily.j.hotton@gmail.com
Zeshan: zeshanqureshi@doctors.org.uk, @DrZeshanQureshi
Facebook: http://www.facebook.com/TheUnofficialGuideToMedicine?fref=ts

FOREWORD

This book is the latest addition to 'The Unofficial Guide to…' series, giving high quality advice and guidance to medical students through their transition into doctors. Previous books in the series have focused on tackling the nuances of OSCE stations. However, 'The Unofficial Guide to Practical Skills' aims to reflect the recent emphasis, by the General Medical Council (GMC), on practical skills.

Approaching practical stations in exams can be challenging. Many medical students struggle to get hands-on experience of practical procedures during time on the wards. In addition, doctors have their own methods for a given skill and contrasting advice can be given. Although a breadth of opinion is good to allow you to develop, it can be a hurdle under exam pressure. This book provides an interactive framework from which to hang this array of knowledge. Directing you through a wide range of scenarios, from knee joint aspirations and ascitic taps to administering oxygen, with skill specific mark schemes, it gives you a clear structure from which to hone and perfect your practical skills.

The once daunting prospect of approaching practical skills can now be overcome by using this refreshingly comprehensive and user-friendly guide. Including both skills focused upon by the GMC and an array of additional skills essential in the armoury of a junior doctor, this book really is the must have!

Best of luck with all your practical skills!

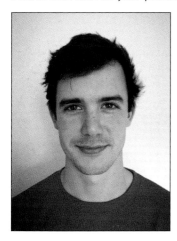

Robert Miller, Final Year Medical Student, University of Bristol

HOW TO USE THIS BOOK

This book has been created for you. **We aim to ease the stress of studying and assist in making learning enjoyable to help you become a better clinician.** The book is split into eight chapters, following a logical order from simple procedures to those that are more challenging.

Each practical skill station has a method outlining how to perform the skill as well as detailed objectives, general advice and facts dispersed throughout. This is followed by a matched mark scheme and a series of questions. This format allows for individual study or group work. There are three roles that may be adopted: the patient; the examiner and the candidate. The roles of the patient and examiner can be combined if working in pairs.

Scenario

These are real life instructions that would be found in OSCEs or on the wards. Take your time to read the passage and note any salient points. In OSCE scenarios you will not be able to ask the examiner any questions regarding the passage, so carefully reading it before starting is paramount.

Mark Scheme

This is a checklist of points that are important to cover in each station. It is not based on any specific university mark scheme, but covers principles we believe are important to address. The examiner can tick off points in the boxes as they are covered. These mark schemes can be used several times to gauge progress over a period of time.

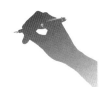

Questions and Answers for Candidate

These questions can be asked to the candidate with model answers provided.

Additional Questions to Consider

These are other questions surrounding the theme of the station. They are ones to consider, discuss and think through further to those provided.

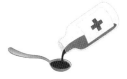

ABBREVIATIONS AND SYMBOLS

o	degrees
ABPI	ankle brachial pressure index
AMD	age-related macular degeneration
ß	beta
BE	base excess
BiPAP	bilevel positive airway pressure
BMI	body mass index
BP	blood pressure
cm	centimetre(s)
cmH_2O	centimetre of water
CO_2	carbon dioxide
COPD	chronic obstructive pulmonary disease
CPAP	continuous positive airway pressure
CPR	cardiopulmonary resuscitation
CRP	C reactive protein
CSF	cerebrospinal fluid
CT	computed tomography
CVP	central venous pressure
DKA	diabetic ketoacidosis
DLCO	diffusion capacity of the lung for carbon monoxide
ECG	electrocardiogram
EDTA	ethylenediaminetetraacetic acid
FBC	full blood count
FEV_1	forced expiratory volume in one second
FiO_2	inspired oxygen concentration
FVC	forced vital capacity
GCS	Glasgow Coma Score
Hb	haemoglobin
HCO_3^-	bicarbonate
HAS	human albumin solution
ICP	intracranial pressure
ID	identification
IJV	internal jugular vein
INR	international normalised ratio
IV	intravenous
kg	kilograms

kPa	kilopascal(s) pressure
L	litre
LA	local anaesthetic
LFTs	liver function tests
LP	lumbar puncture
m	metres
MC&S	microscopy, culture and sensitivity
mg	milligram(s)
MI	myocardial infarction
min	minute(s)
mL	millilitre(s)
mmHg	millimetres of mercury pressure
mmol	millimoles
MRSA	methicillin-resistant Staphylococcus aureus
NPDR	non-proliferative diabetic retinopathy
NTT	non touch technique
O_2	oxygen
OP	oropharyngeal
$PaCO_2$	arterial partial pressure of carbon dioxide
PaO_2	arterial partial pressure of oxygen
PCI	primary coronary intervention
PEA	pulseless electrical activity
PICC	peripherally inserted central catheter
PPE	personal protective equipment
PT	prothrombin time
SaO_2	arterial oxygen saturation
SAAG	serum-ascites albumin gradient
SBP	spontaneous bacterial peritonitis
STEMI	ST elevation myocardial infarction
TB	tuberculosis
TLCO	transfer factor of the lung for carbon monoxide
U&E	urea and electrolyte
USS	ultrasound scan
VF	ventricular fibrillation
VT	ventricular tachycardia
WCC	white cell count

CONTRIBUTORS

Editors

Emily Hotton   Foundation Doctor (University of Bristol)
Zeshan Qureshi   Academic Clinical Fellow - Paediatrics (University of Southampton)

Senior Advisor

Dr Natalie Blencowe   NIHR Doctoral Research Fellow and Honorary Specialty Registrar, Surgery, University of Bristol

Practical Skills Authors

Andiran Anduvan Core Medical Trainee (Charles University, Prague)
Diagnostic Ascitic Tap
ECGs
Otoscopy
Spirometry
Therapeutic Paracentesis

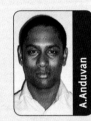

Srikant Ganesh Foundation Doctor (University of Bristol)
Chest Drain
Diagnostic Ascitic Tap
Diagnostic Pleural Tap
Instruments
Proctoscopy
Surgical Gowning and Gloving
Suturing

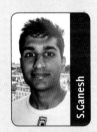

Nikki Hall Opthalmology Trainee (University of Edinburgh)
Fundoscopy

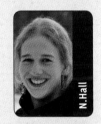

Ruth Harrison Foundation Doctor (University of Bristol)
Death Certification
ECGs
Female Urethral Catheterisation
Fundoscopy
Inhaler Technique
Local Anaesthetic Administration
Male Urethral Catheterisation
Peak Flow

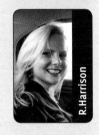

James Hayward Foundation Doctor (University of Bristol)
Administering Oxygen
Airway Management
Central Venous Lines
Immediate Life Support
Intravenous Cannulation
Lumbar Puncture
Setting Up a Giving Set

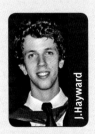

Practical Skills Authors Continued

Emily Hotton Foundation Doctor (University of Bristol)

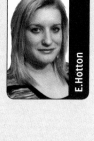

Ankle Brachial Pressure Index
Arterial Blood Gas
Blood Cultures
Blood Glucose
Blood Pressure
Blood Gas Interpretation
Blood Transfusion
Body Mass Index
Choking
Drug Administration via Nebuliser
Hand Washing
Heart Rate and Respiratory Rate
Infection Control
Intradermal Injections
Intramuscular Injections
Intravenous Drugs
Knee Joint Aspiration
Lying and Standing Blood Pressure
Manual Handling
MRSA Swab
Nasogastric Tube Insertion
Nutritional Assessment
Operating a Syringe Driver
Oxygen Saturation
Phlebotomy
Preparing Baby Formula Milk
Simple Dressing Change
Sizing and Fitting a Hard Collar
Subcutaneous Injections
Suprapubic Catheterisation
Urinalysis

Katrina Mason Core Surgical Trainee (University of Bristol)

Suturing

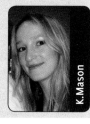

Senior Reviewers

Dr Steven Alderson	National Medical Director's Clinical Fellow to Health Education England
Dr James Andrews	Medical Registrar, Wellington Regional Hospital, NZ
Ken Arber	Clinical Education Facilitator, University Hospitals Southampton
Dr Patrick Byrne	Consultant Physician and GP, Belford Hospital Fort William
Frances Haig	Clinical Education Facilitator, University Hospitals Southampton
Elizabeth Hotton	Sister and Unit Manager, Mount Edgcumbe Hospice, Cornwall
Dr Chris Lang	Consultant Cardiologist, Edinburgh Royal Infirmary, Edinburgh
Sophie Macadie	Clinical Education Facilitator, University Hospitals Southampton
Tracey Murphy	Clinical Education Facilitator, University Hospitals Southampton
Dr David Tate	Gastroenterology Registrar, Royal United Hospital, Bath
Mr Jonathan Wyatt	Emergency Department Consultant, Royal Cornwall Hospital, Truro

Student Reviewers

Alexander Curtis	University of Bristol
Vanessa Hayter	University of Bristol
Amelia Holloway	Peninsula Medical School
Katherine Lattey	Brighton and Sussex Medical School

CONTENTS

Station 2: OXYGEN SATURATION

Mr Michael has just walked back from the toilet and now feels breathless. Please record Mr Michael's oxygen saturation.

Objectives

- Measuring and interpreting oxygen saturation

General Advice

- Always wash your hands before and after patient contact and obtain consent before starting the procedure
- At the end of the procedure, discuss your findings with the patient and record them appropriately in the notes

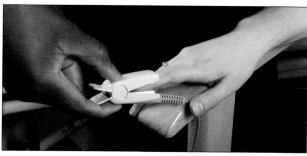
Fig 1.2: Ensure the probe is placed on the finger with the sensor on the dorsal aspect of the hand

Measuring Oxygen Saturation

1. Ensure that the patient is comfortable and select a forefinger that is clean and without nail polish (Fig 1.2)
2. Correctly position the oxygen saturation probe onto the end of the forefinger and ensure the machine is turned on
3. Read off the oxygen saturation
4. Note whether the patient is breathing room air or is receiving supplementary oxygen

It is important to know the target range for a patient's oxygen saturations. In most fit and healthy people, this target range is 94-98%. For some patients, such as those with chronic obstructive pulmonary disease (COPD), their target range may be 88-92%

'Nail polish, fake nails, nicotine staining and insufficient arterial blood flow through the sensor can disrupt the accuracy of oxygen saturation readings. Consider moving the sensor to another site, such as the earlobe, if necessary'

Mark Scheme for Examiner

Introduction and General Preparation

Introduces self (clean hands)

Identifies patient (3 points of ID)

Explains procedure, identifies concerns and obtains consent

Measuring the Oxygen Saturation

Exposes the patient's hand and ensures no nail polish (if applicable)

Checks if the patient is on supplementary oxygen

Positions probe correctly onto finger

Finishing

Documents findings in patient notes

Discusses findings with patient

Questions and Answers for Candidate

Q&A

Additional Questions to Consider

Where can an oxygen probe be placed?

- Finger
- Toe
- Ear lobe

Name two causes of hypoxaemia

- Low concentration of inspired oxygen, e.g. breathing at high altitude
- Right to left shunting (blood bypasses the lungs), e.g. Eisenmenger's syndrome
- Ventilation-perfusion mismatch, e.g. pneumonia, pulmonary oedema
- Diffusion impairment, e.g. interstitial lung disease
- Hypoventilation, e.g. brain stem tumour, intracerebral haemorrhage, Guillain-Barré syndrome

1. How would you assess a patient found to be hypoxaemic?
2. What other investigations would you undertake in a patient found to be hypoxaemic?
3. What are the different ways you might deliver oxygen to a patient?
4. When would you perform an arterial blood gas in a patient with low oxygen saturations?
5. What is the normal range of oxygen saturations, and how would you determine a patient's oxygen saturation target?

Station 3: BLOOD PRESSURE

Mrs Space has recently stopped her anti-hypertensive medication. Please check her blood pressure (BP).

Objectives

- Measuring and interpreting BP using manual and electronic techniques

General Advice

- Always wash your hands before and after patient contact and obtain valid consent before performing the procedure
- At the end of the procedure, discuss your findings with the patient and record them appropriately in the notes
- Ensure that the patient is comfortable and adequately expose the right arm
- Correctly position the arm so it is supported. The point at which you will measure the BP in the arm should be approximately level with the heart
- Select an appropriately sized cuff

For the Manual Technique

1. Correctly place the BP cuff on the patient's arm (Fig 1.3)

'Make sure the patient is not wearing tight sleeves as this can affect the accuracy of blood pressure readings'

2. Locate the brachial artery (usually found at the medial border of the antecubital fossa, medial to the biceps tendon)
3. Inflate the cuff until the pulse becomes impalpable
4. Note the pressure on the manometer

Continues overleaf...

It is important that the BP cuff is correctly sized for your patient. If it is incorrect, your reading may be falsely low or elevated. Most cuffs have sizing marked on them for easy reference. Alternatively, if you are unable to wrap the cuff correctly around the patient's arm, you need to select a different cuff

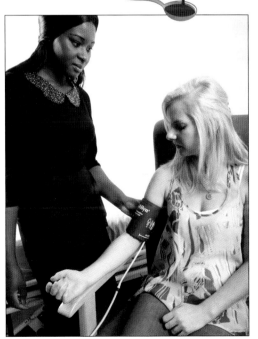

Fig 1.3: The patient's arm should be positioned so it is at the level of the heart

5. Deflate the cuff and place the stethoscope over the brachial artery (Fig 1.4)

6. Re-inflate the cuff to a pressure 20 millimeters of mercury (mmHg) higher than that noted previously

7. Deflate the cuff by 2mmHg per second

8. Note the pressure at which you hear the first heart sounds (systolic blood pressure)

9. Continue to deflate the cuff and note the pressure at which the heart sounds completely disappear (diastolic blood pressure)

For an Automatic Electronic Device

1. Correctly place the blood pressure cuff on the patient's arm

2. Switch on the blood pressure device and press the start button

3. Note the blood pressure reading and document your findings on the patient's observation chart

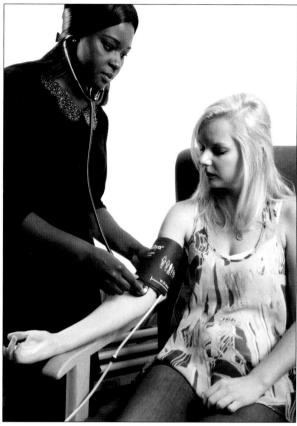

Fig 1.4: Use the stethoscope to determine the systolic and diastolic pressures

Ensure the patient does not talk whilst you are taking the blood pressure. This can not only change the reading, but it will also help you to hear better

Remember!

You cannot make a diagnosis of hypertension from a single high blood pressure reading

Guideline:

Management of Hypertension, World Health Organisation, 2003
http://www.who.int/cardiovascular_diseases/guidelines/hypertension_guidelines.pdf

Mark Scheme for Examiner

Introduction and General Preparation

Introduces self (clean hands)

Identifies patient (3 points of ID)

Explains procedure, identifies concerns and obtains consent

Exposes right arm (or left arm if any issues with using right arm)

Positions arm blood pressure measurement point at the level of the heart

Selects and applies an appropriately sized cuff

Measuring the BP – the Manual Technique

Palpates the brachial artery

Inflates the cuff to systole

Deflates the cuff

Positions the stethoscope

Re-inflates the cuff to 20mmHg above systole

Deflates cuff at the appropriate rate

Notes the systolic and diastolic pressures

Measuring the BP – for Automatic Electronic Device

Switches on the machine and starts the recording

Reads the blood pressure correctly

Finishing

Documents findings in patient notes

Discusses findings with patient

Questions and Answers for Candidate

Additional Questions to Consider

What can make a BP recording inaccurate?

- If the patient is anxious
- If the patient has not adequately rested before the blood pressure reading
- If the BP cuff size is incorrect
- If only one BP reading is taken

In what situations would it be advisable to take the BP from the left arm?

- If the right arm has an intravenous (IV) infusion in situ
- If the right arm is paralysed
- If there is lymphoedema in the right arm
- If there is a fistula in the right arm
- Patient preference

1. How is hypertension diagnosed?

2. What lifestyle advice can be given to patients with high BP?

3. What are the common first-line medications for hypertension?

4. What is malignant hypertension? How is this assessed and managed?

5. How might ethnicity affect choice of medication in treating hypertension?

Station 4: LYING AND STANDING BLOOD PRESSURE

Mrs Monty is a 69 year-old woman who presents to you in the Emergency Department with recurrent falls. Please perform a lying and standing BP and relay your findings.

Objectives

- Performing lying and standing BP
- Interpreting results of lying and standing BP

General Advice

- Lying and standing BP can be used to diagnose (or demonstrate) postural hypotension. Ensure that you have time to perform the examination properly and you are not rushing the patient, as this may falsely elevate their BP reading

Performing Lying and Standing BP

1. Introduce yourself to the patient and obtain valid consent
2. Position the patient supine and ensure that they have been lying there for at least five minutes (Fig 1.5)
3. Take the patient's BP as outlined previously in station 1.3
4. Document the lying systolic and diastolic pressures
5. Leave the cuff in place and ask the patient to stand (Fig 1.6)
6. Inform the patient they need to stand for one minute before you will re-take the BP
7. Ensure the arm is supported at the level of the heart
8. Re-take the BP as outlined previously
9. Remove the cuff and allow the patient to sit
10. Document the standing systolic and diastolic pressures
11. Explain your findings to the patient

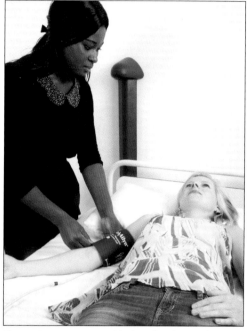

Fig 1.5: Ensure correct positioning of patient and BP cuff

> 'Some patients are unable to tolerate lying flat for long periods of time. Before you ask them to lie flat, ensure that you ask them if they are able to lie flat. If they are unable to lie completely flat, be aware that your examination findings may need to be interpreted with caution. Alternatively, you may wish to pragmatically do a sitting BP instead of a lying BP'

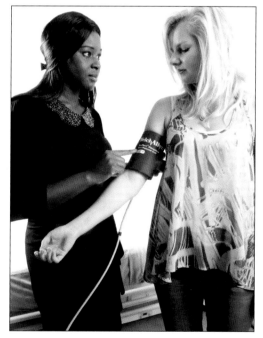

Fig 1.6: The BP cuff can be kept in situ between lying and standing

Present Your Findings

Mrs Monty is a 69 year-old woman who has presented with a fall. On examination her, lying BP was 146/82mmHg and her standing BP was 118/78mmHg. She therefore has a postural systolic drop of greater that 20mmHg, which is suggestive of postural hypotension. I would like to determine the cause of her postural hypotension, so I would take a full history and examine her with a particular focus on the cardiovascular exam and her fluid status. I would also look at the observations chart, and review her current medications.

Mark Scheme for Examiner

Introduction and General Preparation

Introduces self (clean hands)

Identifies patient (3 points of ID)

Explains procedure, identifies concerns and obtains consent

Performing Lying BP

Positions the patient supine

Leaves the patient lying for 5 minutes

Takes the blood pressure

Performing Standing BP

Leaves the cuff in place

Asks the patient to stand

Leaves the patient standing for 1 minute

Re-takes the BP as previously outlined

Finishing

Removes the cuff and allow the patient to sit

Documents findings in patient notes

Discusses findings with patient

Questions and Answers for Candidate

How would you define postural hypotension?

- Postural (or orthostatic) hypotension is defined as a fall in systolic BP >20mmHg or a drop in diastolic BP >10mmHg when a patient assumes a standing position as compared to when they are lying down

Describe the management for a well patient with postural hypotension

- Treat any reversible causes, such as poor fluid intake or medications like antihypertensives
- Conservative measures (e.g. not standing up too quickly)
- Compression bandaging could be considered to improve venous return
- If conservative measures fail, consider specific medication such as fludrocortisone

Additional Questions to Consider

1. What are the signs and symptoms of postural hypotension?
2. What is a tilt table test?
3. How might postural hypotension present?
4. What is postural orthostatic tachycardia syndrome?
5. What are the problems with interpreting lying and standing BPs?

Station 5: ANKLE BRACHIAL PRESSURE INDEX

Mr Fisher is a 68-year-old man who presents to your clinic with pain and cramping in his left lower leg. The pain occurs on walking and is relieved by rest. Mr Fisher is a smoker and is receiving medical treatment for hyperlipidaemia and hypertension. Please measure the Ankle Brachial Pressure Index (ABPI) and tell the examiner your interpretation of the findings

Objectives

* Measuring and interpreting ABPI readings

General Advice

* Make sure that you have protected any ulcers that may be present

Measuring ABPI

1. Introduce yourself to the patient and obtain valid consent
2. Position the patient supine to remove the effect of gravity on blood flow
3. Place an appropriately sized cuff around the right calf
4. Locate the dorsalis pedis or posterior tibial pulse (Fig 1.7)
5. Place the Doppler gel and probe on the skin near to where you expect to find the pulse (Fig 1.8)
6. Listen for the sound of blood flow, a 'whoosh-whoosh' sound
7. Inflate the cuff until the sound of blood flow has disappeared
8. Deflate the cuff by 2mmHg/second until you hear the blood flow returning and note this ankle systolic pressure
9. Place an appropriately sized cuff around the patient's right arm
10. Locate the brachial pulse at the medial border of the antecubital fossa (Fig 1.9)
11. Repeat steps 5-8, noting the brachial systolic pressure
12. Repeat steps 3-11 in the opposite limbs
13. Calculate ABPI = $\dfrac{\text{Ankle Systolic Pressure}}{\text{Brachial Systolic Pressure}}$
14. Explain the significance of ABPI to patient and document findings

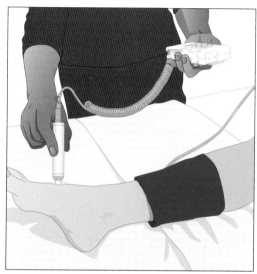

Fig 1.8: Carefully locate the best position to listen to the sound of blood flow with the doppler

'ABPI should always be undertaken before applying a compression bandage to ensure there is not underlying arterial disease'

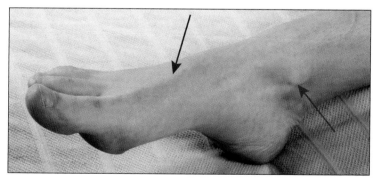

Fig 1.7: Location of the dorsalis pedis (blue arrow) and posterior tibial (red arrow) pulses

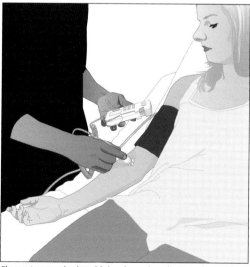

Fig 1.9 Locate the brachial pulse using the Doppler probe

'Patients who have diabetes mellitus or renal failure, or who are heavy smokers, may have falsely high ABPI readings, so findings should be interpreted with caution'

Interpretation of ABPI

ABPI ‹0.5	ABPI 0.5-0.8	ABPI 0.9-1.2	ABPI ›1.3
Indicates severe arterial disease	Indicates moderate arterial disease	Within the normal range	May indicate calcified arteries (and may mask underlying stenosis)

Present Your Findings

Mr Fisher is a 68-year-old man who has presented with intermittent claudication. He has known hypertension and hyperlipidaemia. On examination, his ankle systolic pressure is 80 mmHg and his brachial systolic pressure is 130 mmHg. His ABPI is therefore 0.6; this result, in conjunction with his symptoms, suggests peripheral vascular disease. I would like to take a full history, and examination. He may benefit from referral to the vascular surgeons, and imaging such as an arterial duplex scan.

Mark Scheme for Examiner

Introduction and General Preparation

Introduces self (clean hands)

Identifies patient (3 points of ID)

Explains procedure, identifies concerns and obtains consent

Positions patient supine

Measuring the Ankle Systolic Pressure

Selects and applies an appropriately sized cuff to the calf

Palpates a peripheral pulse

Places the Doppler gel and probe over the artery

Inflates the cuff to above systole

Deflates the cuff

Records the systolic pressure

Measuring the Brachial Systolic Pressure

Selects and applies an appropriately sized cuff to the arm

Palpates the brachial pulse

Places the Doppler gel and probe over the artery

Inflates the cuff to above systole

Deflates the cuff

Records the systolic pressure

Repeat on the opposite limbs

Calculating the ABPI

Correctly calculates the ABPI

Finishing

Wipes any Doppler gel from the patient

Documents findings in patient notes

Discusses findings with patient

Station 9: NUTRITIONAL ASSESSMENT

Mr Moran is a 72-year-old man with dementia from a nursing home. He has been on the ward for several days for the management of pneumonia and a urinary tract infection. Your registrar has asked you to perform a nutritional assessment.

Objectives

- Using the Malnutrition Universal Screening Tool (MUST)
- Managing malnutrition

General Advice

- Obtain valid consent
- Explain to the patient about the questions you are about to ask them
- Use the MUST to assess the patient's nutrition
- In this case, the patient has dementia so you may need to speak to family and other healthcare professionals to obtain the information you require

MUST Screening Tool

Step 1: Calculate BMI		Step 2: Weight loss score		Step 3: Acute disease effect score	
0	BMI >20 kg/m²	0	<5% unplanned weight loss in the past 3-6 months	2	If the patient has been acutely ill and there has been no nutritional intake for >5 days
1	BMI 18.5-20 kg/m²	1	5-10% unplanned weight loss in the past 3-6 months		
2	BMI <18.5 kg/m²	2	>10% unplanned weight loss in the past 3-6 months		

Step 4: Overall risk of malnutrition

Add the scores of step 1, step 2 and step 3 together:

0 = Low Risk	1 = Medium Risk	≥2 = High Risk
Repeat MUST weekly Weigh weekly	Start nutrition action plan Repeat MUST weekly Weigh weekly	Refer to dietician PLUS As for medium risk

Managing Problems with Nutrition

Simple Measures

- Refer to dietician
- Ensure the medical team is aware of patients with nutritional problems
- Follow trust protocol for managing patients with nutritional problems

Dietary Supplementation

- High energy drinks
- Full fat milk
- Multivitamins

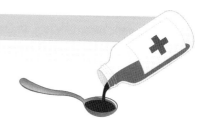

Alternative methods of feeding

Nasogastric (NG) tube feeding	Indicated in those who cannot eat or drink normally by mouth (e.g. those with an 'unsafe' swallow)
Total parenteral nutrition (IV feeding)	Indicated when the gastrointestinal tract is non-functional (such as short bowel syndrome)

Guideline:
Malnutrition Universal Screening Tool, BAPEN, 2011   http://www.bapen.org.uk/pdfs/must/must_full.pdf

BASIC PATIENT ASSESSMENTS

Mark Scheme for Examiner

Introduction and General Preparation

Introduces self (clean hands) ☐ ☐ ☐ ☐ ☐

Identifies patient (3 points of ID) ☐ ☐ ☐ ☐ ☐

Explains procedure, identify concerns and obtains consent ☐ ☐ ☐ ☐ ☐

Assessing Nutrition Status

Calculates BMI ☐ ☐ ☐ ☐ ☐

Discusses any weight loss (and, if appropriate, the time frame) ☐ ☐ ☐ ☐ ☐

Discusses acute disease and nutritional intake ☐ ☐ ☐ ☐ ☐

Calculates risk of malnutrition ☐ ☐ ☐ ☐ ☐

Finishing

Documents findings in patient notes ☐ ☐ ☐ ☐ ☐

Discusses findings with patient ☐ ☐ ☐ ☐ ☐

Questions and Answers for Candidate

Give four risk factors that can predispose to malnutrition

- Swallowing problems, e.g. stroke/motor neurone disease
- Psychological disease, e.g. depression, dementia
- Malabsorption, e.g. coeliac disease, inflammatory bowel disease
- Chronic illness, e.g. COPD resulting in increased energy demands
- Lack of education, learning difficulties or poor access to food
- Acute illness: resulting in increased energy demands and often reduced oral intake

Additional Questions to Consider

1. What investigations would you consider undertaking in a patient who is malnourished?
2. How would you manage a malnourished patient?
3. Which other healthcare professionals would you include in the management of a malnourished patient apart from doctors?
4. What are the complications of being malnourished?
5. What are the two classic clinical presentations of protein malnutrition? Explain the difference between them.

Station 1: PHLEBOTOMY

Mr Frederick is a 50-year-old man who is attending your clinic for a repeat blood test to check his haemoglobin, having recently been in hospital and received a blood transfusion. Please explain to him what you are going to do, and then demonstrate how you would take blood on the mannequin provided.

Objectives

- To learn the correct techniques for phlebotomy
- To learn the common blood tests and draw order

General Advice

- Check patient identification and obtain valid consent
- Check whether the patient has any allergies
- Check whether the patient is needle phobic
- Check for any issues that may affect selection of the site of phlebotomy, e.g. whether they have lymphoedema or an AV fistula, or have had a mastectomy

Equipment Checklist

(remember to check expiry dates on all equipment) (Fig 2.1)

a)   Tray: either single-use, disposable sterilised tray, or a decontaminated plastic tray that is cleaned pre/post procedure

b)   Single use disposable apron

c)   Non-sterile gloves

d)   Disposable tourniquet

e)   Skin cleansing solution [2% chlorhexidine (CHG) and 70% isopropyl alcohol (IPA) (e.g. ChloraPrep®)]

f)   Venepuncture needle

g)   Vacutainer™

h)   Blood bottles

i)   Cotton wool

j)   Tape

k)   Sharps bin: the sharps bin should always be taken to the point of care

Note: Skin cleansing solutions and method with vary depending on local policy. If taking blood cultures, blood culture bottle ports will need to be fully cleaned and allowed to fully dry before use

Explaining the Procedure to the Patient

1.   We need to take a blood sample

2.   We need to put a tight band around your arm to 'bring up' the vein

3.   A small needle is placed into one of your veins in the arm

4.   It will be slightly painful

5.   A blood sample will then be taken

6.   It is possible the doctor may be unable to take a blood sample at the first attempt. If this happens the doctor will ask your permission before trying again

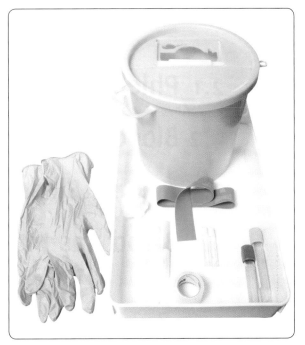

Fig 2.1: Ensure you have all the equipment you require before heading to the bedside

Performing the Procedure
Preparation

1.   Wash hands

2.   Obtain all equipment that may be needed

3.   Assemble equipment:
- Attach Vacutainer™ to venepuncture needle
- Place blood bottles in draw order
- Cut a piece of tape to size

Drawing Blood

1. Clean hands, don non-sterile gloves and apply a single-use disposable apron (Fig 2.2)
2. Place the tourniquet 7-10 cm proximal to the proposed insertion point (Fig 2.3)
3. Select the vein: the vein should feel 'bouncy' – if not, it is either inadequately filled or, if rigid, it may be thrombosed
4. Loosen tourniquet
5. Clean site – clean for 30 seconds with ChloraPrep® in an up-and-down, back-and-forth friction technique. Allow to completely dry (Fig 2.4)
6. Retighten tourniquet. Attach venepuncture needle to Vacutainer™
7. Puncture the vein using a non-touch technique (NTT), warning the patient of a 'sharp scratch' (Fig 2.5)
8. Draw blood by attaching bottles to Vacutainer™. Invert bottles
9. Release tourniquet
10. Immediately dispose of sharps (Fig 2.6)
11. Apply pressure to the puncture site with cotton wool for two minutes or until bleeding stops
12. Secure with tape (Fig 2.7)
13. Label the bottles at the bedside (Fig 2.8)
14. Inform the patient to let a member of staff know if the site is painful, continues to bleed, or if they have any other concerns
15. Explain that they can remove the dressing after a couple of hours

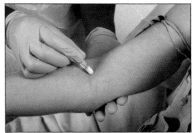
Fig 2.4: Ensure skin is clean

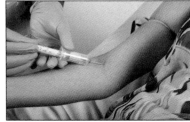
Fig 2.5: Make sure you collect blood in the order of draw

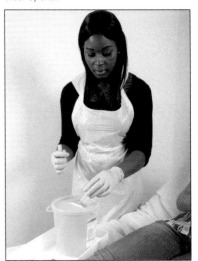
Fig 2.6: Take the sharps bin to the bedside with you

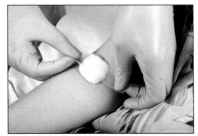
Fig 2.7: Ask the patient to apply pressure, if they are able to

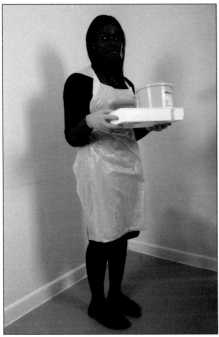
Fig 2.2: Correctly prepare for the procedure using appropriate protective equipment

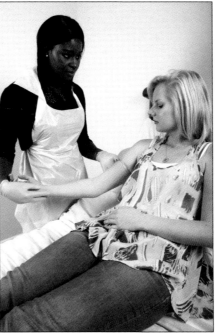
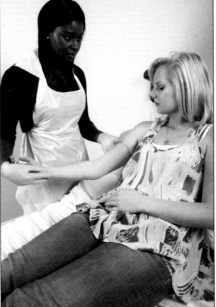
Fig 2.3: Ensure the tourniquet is away from the sterile field

'It is often easier to approach a vein at the junction where two veins join'

Finishing

1. Dispose of equipment
2. Clean the tray
3. Dispose of gloves and wash your hands
4. Send the samples to the pathology labs

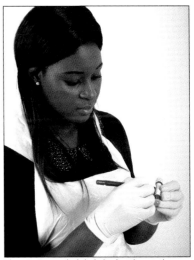
Fig 2.8: Correctly label the bottles at the bedside

Blood Bottles

(In Order of Draw: note, colours may vary between hospitals)

Tube	Colour/Additive	What it can measure	Number of times to invert
Blood cultures	Blue (aerobic) – 5 millilitre (mL) Purple (anaerobic) – 5 mL	Blood culture and sensitivity	3-4 times
Light blue	Sodium citrate – 2.7 mL	INR, PT, APPT	3-4 times
Red	Plain – 10 mL	Hepatitis status, Rubella Serology, Virology, CA125, Coeliac Screen	5-6 times
Gold	SST – 5 mL	TFTs, LFTs, Hormones, Lipids/Triglycerides, Cholesterol, U&E's, CK, Digoxin levels, Paracetamol levels, PSA, βhCG, Haematinics, Amylase	5-6 times
Green	Lithium heparin – 6 mL	Amino Acids, Cortisol, PTH	8-10 times
Lavender	EDTA – 3 mL	FBC, HbA1c, HLA-B27, Cyclosporine, ESR	8-10 times
Pink	EDTA – 6 mL	Group and Save, Cross Match, Blood Group	8-10 times
Grey	Fluoride Oxalate – 2 mL	Glucose, Ethanol	8-10 times
Royal Blue	EDTA – 5 mL	Trace Elements: Zinc, Copper, Selenium, Manganese, Lead	8-10 times

'Always fill the coagulation bottle right up to the line: it won't get processed otherwise!'

Mark Scheme for Examiner

Introduction and General Advice

Introduces self (clean hands) ☐ ☐ ☐ ☐ ☐

Identifies patient (3 points of ID) ☐ ☐ ☐ ☐ ☐

Explains procedure, identify concerns and obtain consent ☐ ☐ ☐ ☐ ☐

Checks for allergies and needle phobia, and any contraindictions to use of left or right arm ☐ ☐ ☐ ☐ ☐

Preparation

Obtains equipment and checks expiry dates ☐ ☐ ☐ ☐ ☐

Applies single use apron ☐ ☐ ☐ ☐ ☐

Washes hands and dons non-sterile gloves ☐ ☐ ☐ ☐ ☐

Assembles equipment ☐ ☐ ☐ ☐ ☐

Drawing Blood

Applies disposable tourniquet ☐ ☐ ☐ ☐ ☐

Chooses an appropriate vein and loosen the tourniquet ☐ ☐ ☐ ☐ ☐

Cleans puncture site and retightens tourniquet ☐ ☐ ☐ ☐ ☐

Warns patient ☐ ☐ ☐ ☐ ☐

Punctures vein and obtains sample ☐ ☐ ☐ ☐ ☐

Selects correct draw order (if applicable) ☐ ☐ ☐ ☐ ☐

Removes tourniquet ☐ ☐ ☐ ☐ ☐

Removes needle and applies pressure ☐ ☐ ☐ ☐ ☐

Disposes of sharp immediately ☐ ☐ ☐ ☐ ☐

Applies dressing over puncture site ☐ ☐ ☐ ☐ ☐

Finishing

Tells patient to inform staff if site becomes painful or continues to bleed and that they can remove the dressing after a few hours ☐ ☐ ☐ ☐ ☐

Labels blood bottles at the bedside ☐ ☐ ☐ ☐ ☐

Disposes of equipment and cleans tray ☐ ☐ ☐ ☐ ☐

Removes gloves and wash hands ☐ ☐ ☐ ☐ ☐

Sends blood samples to pathology lab ☐ ☐ ☐ ☐ ☐

General Points

Talks throughout the procedure to the patient ☐ ☐ ☐ ☐ ☐

Avoids patient contamination (i.e. NTT) ☐ ☐ ☐ ☐ ☐

Questions and Answers for Candidate

What is the order of draw for full blood count (FBC), urea and electrolytes (U&Es) and clotting?

1. Clotting
2. U&E
3. FBC

Give some causes of hyperkalaemia

- Drugs (e.g. potassium sparing diuretics, ACE inhibitors)
- Renal insufficiency (both acute and chronic renal disease may cause hyperkalaemia)
- Diabetic ketoacidosis
- Burns
- Rhabdomyolysis
- Aldosterone deficiency
- Addisonian crises
- Metabolic acidosis

What additives are found in the different blood tubes?

- Full Blood Count: ethylenediaminetetraacetic acid (EDTA)
- Clotting: citrate
- Plasma analysis: lithium heparin (or sodium heparin)
- Glucose: potassium oxalate and sodium fluoride
- Serum tube: no additive, because you want the blood to clot and to centrifuge the serum

Additional Questions to Consider

1. What is D-dimer and when might you request it?
2. What ways can clotting be measured, and what do the different tests represent?
3. What is adjusted calcium or corrected calcium and how is it calculated?
4. How might a full blood count help you differentiate between a bacterial and a viral infection?
5. What is creatinine kinase and when would you request it?

Compensation

When there has been deviation from the normal blood pH, the body activates pathways to try to compensate for the deviation and attempts to bring the pH back within the normal range
- The lungs compensate for a metabolic disturbance by altering the levels of carbon dioxide – this is generally rapid and can occur within minutes
- The kidneys compensate for a respiratory disturbance by controlling the levels of bicarbonate ions – this is generally slower and takes from a few days to a week to occur

A patient can be uncompensated – this usually implies an acute event, the body has not had time to adapt to the change in pH

A patient can be partially compensated – this implies the pH is out of the normal range and the body is making an attempt to compensate for the disturbance. For example, there may be a respiratory acidosis (raised carbon dioxide), and a small metabolic alkalosis (raised bicarbonate) to compensate. However, the compensation is only partial, and therefore the patient remains acidotic

A patient can be fully compensated – the implies the pH is now within the normal range but other values are still abnormal in order to correct the underlying disturbance. This implies a chronic process

Assessing Oxygenation and Ventilation

Why is it important to look at the PaO₂?
The PaO₂ gives an indication of oxygen uptake. When assessing the PaO₂, it is vital to consider the PaCO₂ at the same time

Respiratory Failure: Type 1 - Failure to oxygenate
Characterised by: PaO₂ < 8 kPa and PaCO₂ = normal/low

Respiratory Failure: Type 2 - Failure to ventilate
Characterised by: PaO₂ < 8 kPa and PaCO₂ > 6 kPa

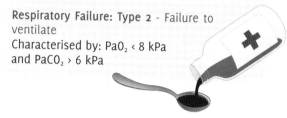

Note: It is important to remember that, in general, overcompensation does not happen; the body brings the pH back within the normal range

Assessing Other Analytes

An arterial sample can provide a **rapid indication** of important analytes such as potassium, haemoglobin and lactate. This can assist in diagnosis and guide early intervention. These can also be obtained from a venous blood gas

Worked Examples

Example 1

pH 7.28	Is the pH acidotic or alkalotic?	Acidotic
PaCO₂ 8.1	Is the pH explained by the PaCO₂?	YES
HCO₃⁻ 25	Is the pH explained by the HCO₃⁻?	NO
	Is there evidence of compensation?	NO
		• The HCO₃⁻ levels are normal
		• The pH is abnormal (so no evidence of full compensation)

Interpretation:
Respiratory acidosis with no compensation
(e.g. more likely an acute change)

Request No:	24891022	Patient No:	4616
Date:	27.11.2013	DOB:	27.03.1959
Time:	01:48		

At 37°C		Arterial Ref Range
pH.............	7.28	7.35-7.45
pCO₂..........	8.1	4.7-6.0
pO₂............	12.2	10.6-13.3
FiO₂...........	0.21	
Cl⁻.............	100	95-105
Na.............	142	135-145
K...............	3.3	3.5-5.0
HCO₃⁻........	25	22-28

Fig 2.16: Example 1

Example 2

pH 7.48	Is the pH acidotic or alkalotic?	Alkalotic
PaCO$_2$ 8.4	Is the pH explained by the PaCO$_2$?	NO
HCO$_3^-$ 38	Is the pH explained by the HCO$_3^-$?	YES
	Is there evidence of compensation?	YES
		• The PaCO$_2$ levels are abnormal (implying compensation)
		• The pH is abnormal (so no evidence of full compensation)

Interpretation:
Metabolic alkalosis with partial respiratory compensation

Example 3

pH 7.30	Is the pH acidotic or alkalotic?	Acidotic
PaCO$_2$ 4.1	Is the pH explained by the PaCO$_2$?	NO
HCO$_3^-$ 18	Is the pH explained by the HCO$_3^-$?	YES
	Is there evidence of compensation?	YES
		• The PaCO$_2$ levels are abnormal (implying compensation)
		• The pH is abnormal (so no evidence of full compensation)

Calculating the anion gap:
$(K^+ 4.2 + Na^+ 134) - (HCO_3^- 18 + Cl^- 102) = 18.2$

Interpretation:
Metabolic acidosis with partial compensation and a increased anion gap

Mr Bridge's Results

pH 7.36	Is the pH acidotic or alkalotic?	Normal (but almost acidotic)
PaCO$_2$ 7.9	Is the pH explained by the PaCO$_2$?	YES (as pH almost classified as acidotic)
HCO$_3^-$ 34	Is the pH explained by the HCO$_3^-$?	NO
	Is there evidence of compensation?	YES
		• The HCO$_3^-$ levels are abnormal (implying compensation)
		• The pH is normal (so evidence of full compensation)
PaO$_2$ 6.8	Is the PaO$_2$ within the normal range?	NO
		• The PaO$_2$ is low indicating hypoxaemia

Interpretation:
Borderline respiratory acidosis with full metabolic compensation and concurrent hypoxia. Putting it all together, most likely chronic type 2 respiratory failure with renal compensation

Request No:	60350029	Patient No:	149
Date:	20.12.2013	DOB:	21.08.1971
Time:	07.51		

At 37°C		Arterial Ref Range
pH	7.48	7.35-7.45
pCO$_2$	8.4	4.7-6.0
pO$_2$	11.8	10.6-13.3
FiO$_2$	0.21	
Cl$^-$	101	95-105
Na	136	135-145
K	4.2	3.5-5.0
HCO$_3^-$	38	22-28

Fig 2.17: Example 2

Request No:	6036781	Patient No:	8912
Date:	20.02.2014	DOB:	01.04.1939
Time:	13.56		

At 37°C		Arterial Ref Range
pH	7.30	7.35-7.45
pCO$_2$	4.1	4.7-6.0
pO$_2$	13.2	10.6-13.3
FiO$_2$	0.21	
Cl$^-$	102	95-105
Na	134	135-145
K	4.2	3.5-5.0
HCO$_3^-$	18	22-28

Fig 2.18: Example 3

Request No:	12569028	Patient No:	3337
Date:	01.10.2013	DOB:	06.08.1956
Time:	09.03		

At 37°C		Arterial Ref Range
pH	7.36	7.35-7.45
pCO$_2$	7.9	4.7-6.0
pO$_2$	6.8	10.6-13.3
FiO$_2$	0.21	
Cl	98	95-105
Na	136	135-145
K	4.0	3.5-5.0
HCO$_3^-$	34	22-28

Fig 2.19: Mr Bridge's ABG results

Station 1: IMMEDIATE LIFE SUPPORT

You are working on a busy Gastroenterology ward when you come across an unresponsive patient in one of the side-rooms. Approach this manikin as you would the patient and perform resuscitation as necessary. Follow any instructions that are given by the examiners during this station.

Objectives

- To recognise a patient in cardiac arrest
- To be able to perform immediate life support
- To know the treatment algorithms for shockable and non-shockable rhythms

Basic Life Support

- Immediate life support is commonly tested with the use of a resuscitation manikin
- It is crucially important to use a systematic approach when dealing with any critically ill patient
- DRS ABC is a useful and well-known mnemonic that will allow you to initiate basic adult life support in a systematic and structured manner

Danger

1. Your own safety is vital – look out for any hazards that might put you at risk. Ask: is it safe to approach?

Response

1. Shake the dummy lightly and shout, 'Hello, can you hear me?', whilst applying a painful stimulus

Shout

1. Shout for help in the event of an unresponsive patient

Airway

1. If there is no concern about a spinal injury, perform a head tilt, chin lift manoeuvre (Fig 3.1)
2. Clear the mouth of any obstruction or foreign body if confident that the object can be removed
3. Use of suction apparatus or repositioning the patient on their side may help (Fig 3.2)

Breathing & Circulation

Simultaneously (whilst maintaining the chin lift):

LOOK for chest movement for 10 seconds

LISTEN for breath sounds for 10 seconds

FEEL the carotid pulse for 10 seconds

In clinical practice, if in doubt, call the crash team and start cardiopulmonary resuscitation (CPR)

- You should proceed to chest compressions immediately, provided that you are confident further help is on the way. Within hospital, this means putting out a crash call via the switchboard. Send a colleague to perform this if it has not been done already, giving the details of the clinical scenario (adult cardiac arrest) and your location (ward)
- Ask your colleague to bring back the crash trolley on their return – this will contain vital resuscitation equipment

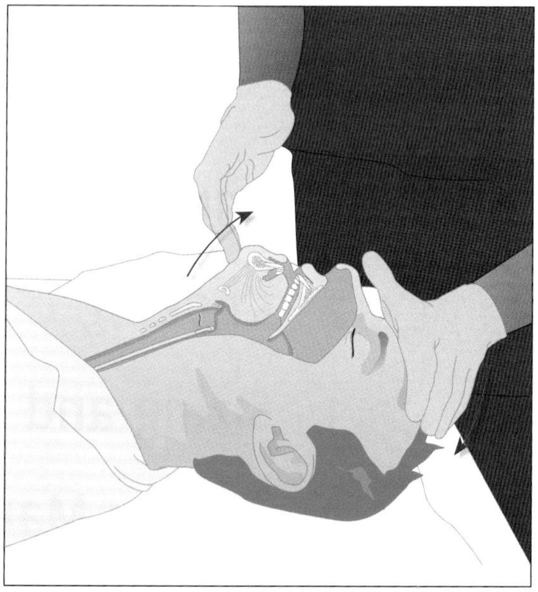

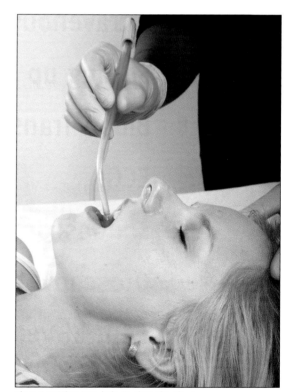

Fig 3.1: This simple action can sometimes be enough to open an airway

Fig 3.2: Suction may help to clear the airway

Success of the resuscitation attempt is highly dependent on prompt defibrillation, as well as high quality CPR and timely arrival of the crash team. Therefore, if you are alone with a patient that you believe is in cardiac arrest and no one responds to your shouts for help, leave the bedside in order to call the cardiac arrest team and obtain the crash trolley

Chest Compressions

1. Start chest compressions;

    POSITION: directly over the bottom half of the sternum (Fig 3.3)

    RATE: 100 –120/minute (min)

    DEPTH: 1/3 of the depth of the chest. In most adults this equates to 5-6cm

2. After 30 compressions, give two breaths using a bag valve mask device connected to high flow oxygen (15L/min). Make sure you maintain a patent airway, otherwise bag valve ventilation will not work. (Fig 3.4) The use of airway adjuncts may be required

3. Continue compressions and breaths at a rate of 30:2

Defibrillation

1. Ask your colleague to proceed with the chest compressions and ventilation breaths

2. Turn on the defibrillator and apply the self-adhesive defibrillation/monitoring pads (ensure that you familiarise yourself with the defibrillators in local use)

> 'The defibrillator pads contain electrodes for determining cardiac rhythm and are quick to apply — do not waste time attaching ECG electrodes if they are not already on the patient'

3. One pad is placed below the right clavicle, the second is placed in the V6 position in the midaxillary line on the left (Fig 3.5)

4. Ensure that chest compressions continue whilst the pads are sited

5. Once the pads are connected, charge defibrillator, asking all (except the person performing CPR) to stand clear. Ensure oxygen is moved away. Once charged, ask your helper to stop CPR so that you can assess the rhythm on the defibrillator display (Fig 3.6)

6. The principal purpose of the rhythm check is to determine whether it is SHOCKABLE or NON-SHOCKABLE

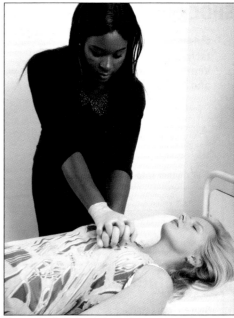

Fig 3.3: Use both hands to perform compressions on an adult

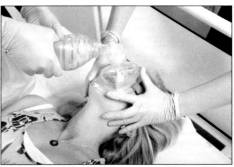

Fig 3.4: If possible, use two people to operate a bag valve mask

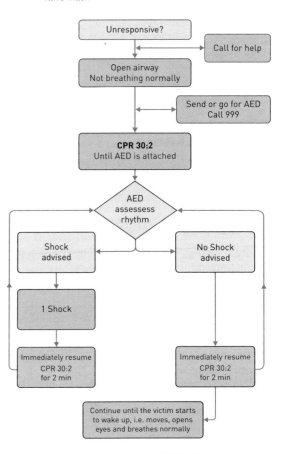

Fig 3.7: Resuscitation Council (UK) AED Algorithm (automated external defibrillator)

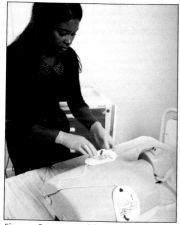

Fig 3.5: Correct position of the pads is important

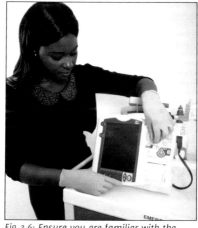

Fig 3.6: Ensure you are familiar with the defibrillator used in your trust

Mark Scheme for Examiner

General
Washes hands   ☐ ☐ ☐ ☐ ☐

Puts on non-sterile gloves   ☐ ☐ ☐ ☐ ☐

Airway Maneuvers
Performs 'head tilt, chin lift' correctly   ☐ ☐ ☐ ☐ ☐

Performs 'jaw thrust' correctly   ☐ ☐ ☐ ☐ ☐

Airway Adjuncts
Correctly identifies oropharyngeal airway   ☐ ☐ ☐ ☐ ☐

Chooses appropriate size for mannequin   ☐ ☐ ☐ ☐ ☐

Correct insertion technique   ☐ ☐ ☐ ☐ ☐

Correctly identifies nasopharyngeal airway   ☐ ☐ ☐ ☐ ☐

Chooses appropriate size for mannequin   ☐ ☐ ☐ ☐ ☐

Correct insertion technique   ☐ ☐ ☐ ☐ ☐

Advanced Airway (LMA)
Correctly identifies LMA   ☐ ☐ ☐ ☐ ☐

Prepares LMA for insertion   ☐ ☐ ☐ ☐ ☐

Correct insertion technique   ☐ ☐ ☐ ☐ ☐

Checks positioning by assessing breath sounds/chest wall movements   ☐ ☐ ☐ ☐ ☐

General Points
Talks clearly to the examiner throughout the station   ☐ ☐ ☐ ☐ ☐

Remains calm and works methodically   ☐ ☐ ☐ ☐ ☐

Questions and Answers for Candidate

When should the 'head tilt, chin lift' manoeuvre not be performed?

- Whenever there is a suspicion of possible cervical spine injury

What is the most important contraindication to nasopharyngeal airway insertion?

- Basal skull fracture

Additional Questions to Consider

1. What re-positioning techniques might be used in patients with known cervical spine injury?

2. What other equipment would you expect to find in the 'Airway' drawer of a crash trolley?

3. What equipment is required to perform intubation?

4. What types of patients would prompt you to anticipate difficulty in airway management?

5. What is the difference between a secure and a non secure airway?

Station 5: ADMINISTERING OXYGEN

You are a junior doctor working in the Emergency Department when Mr Hill, a 62-year-old man, presents acutely short of breath. A nurse performs a set of basic observations, which reveal his oxygen saturations to be 85%. You decide this patient requires supplementary oxygen therapy. What methods for delivering oxygen are available and which might be most appropriate in this situation?

Objectives

- Be aware of the various methods available for delivering supplementary oxygen
- Be able to determine which method is most appropriate for a given scenario

General Advice

- There are several ways in which supplementary oxygen can be delivered
- Titrate the oxygen you administer according to the patient's oxygen saturations
- As with medications, oxygen should be prescribed on a drug chart

Nasal cannulae – the stable patient

- Nasal cannulae consist of a length of oxygen tubing with two nasal prongs, and are looped over the ears and beneath the chin (Fig 3.29)
- Typically preferred by the patient for comfort
- Beware:
  - The amount of oxygen delivered is variable and imprecise
  - Nasal soreness or epistaxis may arise from higher flow rates or prolonged use
  - Achievable flow rate: 1-4L/min
  - Achievable FiO_2: 24-40%

Simple mask – the acutely ill patient

- A transparent facemask with an oxygen tubing connector and elasticised strap
- Less comfortable than nasal cannulae (Fig 3.30)
- Beware:
  - Must be used with flow rate of 5-10L/min (if less that 5L is used, excessive levels of CO_2 can accumulate within the mask)
  - These masks should be avoided in patients at risk of type 2 respiratory failure (see box)
  - Achievable flow rate: 5-10L/min
  - Achievable FiO_2: 40-60%

Respiratory Failure: Type 1

- Failure to oxygenate
- PaO_2 <8kPa
- $PaCO_2$ = normal/low

Respiratory Failure: Type 2

- Failure to ventilate
- PaO_2 <8kPa
- $PaCO_2$ >6kPa

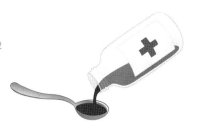

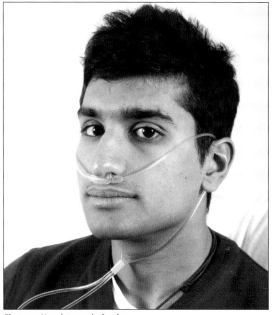

Fig 3.29: Nasal cannula in situ

The 'flow rate' refers to the value you should adjust the oxygen wall outlet to e.g. 10L/min or 5L/min

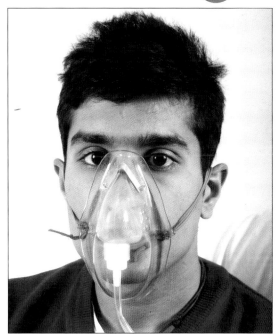

Fig 3.30: Simple facemask in situ

Due to long-standing hypercapnia, patients in type 2 respiratory failure may have a hypoxia-driven respiratory centre. Care should be taken in administering oxygen to these patients as administering too much will cause them to become apnoeic. Start with a Venturi facemask FiO$_2$ 24-28% and aim for target saturations of 88-92%; make sure the nursing staff are aware of this target range

Venturi masks – the acutely ill patient who may develop type II respiratory failure (e.g. known COPD)

- Similar in appearance to the simple facemask but with the addition of a specially designed (and colour-coded) adapter allowing a precise FiO$_2$ to be administered
- For use when it is crucially important to deliver a fixed and specific FiO$_2$ (i.e. in Type 2 respiratory failure) (Fig 3.31)
- Beware:
    o You must ensure that you select the correct adapter for your patient, and review their oxygen saturations regularly
    o Achievable flow rate: dependent on the colour-coded adapter (see below)
    o Achievable FiO$_2$: 24-60% (see below)

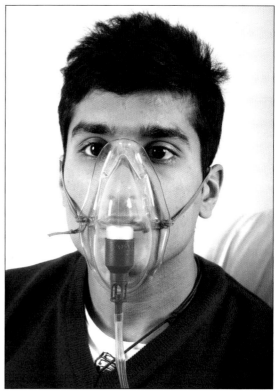

Fig 3.31: Venturi facemask in situ

Possible FiO$_2$ that may be achieved using the Venturi facemask:

60% (12 L/min)   GREEN
40% (10 L/min)   RED
35% (8 L/min)   YELLOW
28% (4 L/min)   WHITE
24% (2 L/min)   BLUE

Non-rebreather mask – the critically ill patient

- Non-rebreather masks comprise a facemask plus reservoir bag
- By using a high flow rate, a reservoir bag can deliver a high FiO$_2$ (Fig 3.32)
- The reservoir bag needs to be filled with air before use
- Beware:
    o The use of a non-rebreather mask is not recommended in patients who require precisely controlled O$_2$ delivery
    o Often used in emergency or trauma situations
    o Achievable flow rate: 10-15L/min
    o Achievable FiO$_2$: 60-90%

FiO$_2$
This is the fraction or percentage of oxygen in the space being measured. Natural air contains 21% oxygen, which correlates to a FiO$_2$ of 0.21

PaO$_2$
This is the partial pressure of oxygen gas, dissolved in the blood. This can only be measured by performing an arterial blood gas analysis

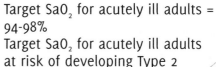

Target SaO$_2$ for acutely ill adults = 94-98%
Target SaO$_2$ for acutely ill adults at risk of developing Type 2 respiratory failure = 88-92%

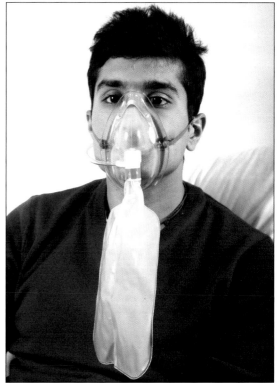

Fig 3.32: Non-rebeather mask in situ

'An arterial blood gas provides the PaO_2, which can both be helpful in terms of planning how to deliver oxygen and to determine how much to provide. Therefore, arterial blood gas should ALWAYS be considered when you are asked to review a patient who is experiencing breathing difficulties'

Mark Scheme for Examiner

Nasal Cannulae

Correctly identifies equipment	☐	☐	☐	☐	☐
Describes correct method of application	☐	☐	☐	☐	☐
States that these are for use in a stable patient	☐	☐	☐	☐	☐
States correct achievable flow rates (1-4L/min) and FiO_2 (24-40%)	☐	☐	☐	☐	☐

Simple Facemask

Correctly identifies equipment	☐	☐	☐	☐	☐
Describes correct method of application	☐	☐	☐	☐	☐
States that this is for use in an acutely ill patient	☐	☐	☐	☐	☐
States correct achievable flow rates (5-10L/min) and FiO_2 (40-60%)	☐	☐	☐	☐	☐

Venturi Mask

Correctly identifies equipment	☐	☐	☐	☐	☐
Describes correct method of application	☐	☐	☐	☐	☐
States that this is for use in an acutely ill patient when a precise FiO_2 is required	☐	☐	☐	☐	☐
Mentions type II respiratory failure or COPD as appropriate indications	☐	☐	☐	☐	☐
States that there are a range of colour-coded adaptors to be used with various flow rates in order to achieve different FiO_2 values	☐	☐	☐	☐	☐

Non-rebreather Mask

Correctly identifies equipment	☐	☐	☐	☐	☐
Describes correct method of application and the need to fill reservoir bag	☐	☐	☐	☐	☐
States that this is for use in a critically ill patient	☐	☐	☐	☐	☐
States correct achievable flow rates (10-15L/min) and FiO_2 (60-90%)	☐	☐	☐	☐	☐

General Points

Talks clearly to the examiner throughout the station	☐	☐	☐	☐	☐

Questions and Answers for Candidate

What would be the most appropriate method for use in the case of Mr Hill?

- A non-rebreather facemask with high flow oxygen (10-15L/min) provided he has no underlying lung pathology contraindicating high flow oxygen

Why is high-flow oxygen potentially problematic in patients with type II respiratory failure?

- Due to long-standing hypercapnia, these patients may have a hypoxia-driven respiratory centre. High-flow oxygen could suppress this drive, resulting in apnoea

Additional Questions to Consider

1. How would you differentiate type I and type II respiratory failure, on the basis of ABG results?
2. What patient information must you take into account when prescribing oxygen?
3. What are the indications for non-invasive ventilation?
4. Describe the difference between bilevel positive airway pressure (BiPAP) and continuous positive airway pressure (CPAP) ventilation
5. Outline some causes of hypoxia

Station 6: INTRAVENOUS CANNULATION

Mrs Jones has been diagnosed with small bowel obstruction. She requires cannulation so that IV fluids can be administered. Please obtain consent for this and then, on the mannequin provided, demonstrate how to insert an IV cannula.

Objectives

- To learn correct technique for cannula insertion

General Advice

- Obtain valid consent
- Ask the patient if they have an arm preference
- Consider if there are any pre-disposing medical or surgical conditions that would not allow using a specific arm/blood vessel, such as a renal fistula, cellulitis, mastectomy
- Check if the patient has any allergies such as to chlorhexidine

Equipment Checklist

(remember to check expiry dates on all equipment) (Fig 3.33)

a) Skin cleansing solution (e.g. ChloraPrep®)
b) 21-gauge needle (though for drawing up medications, IN ALL cases a blunt draw up needle is preferred if available)
c) 10 mL syringe and syringe cap (or second needle if syringe cap not available)
d) 10 mL 0.9% saline ampoule for flush
e) Sterile adhesive dressing
f) Cannula
g) Disposable tourniquet
h) Cotton wool
i) 2 pairs of non-sterile gloves
j) Tape (if you fail to site the cannula you will need to tape some cotton wool over the puncture site)
k) Tray (as with phlebotomy)
l) Sharps bin: the sharps bin should always be taken to the point of care
m) Single use disposable apron

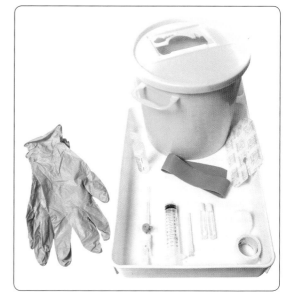

Fig 3.33: Equipment required for cannulation

'If the patient has suffered vasovagal episodes with needles in the past, lay the patient flat'

Note: Skin-cleansing methods and methods of capping will vary depending on local policy. In addition, local policy may use alternative methods to cap. Any tubing that is attached, such as a bioconnector or a line, needs to be flushed first with 0.9% saline to avoid injecting air and risking an air embolus

Cannulae are sized by gauge (smaller the number = bigger the size), all with corresponding colours. Bigger cannulae can achieve higher flow rates. For administering IV medication and IV maintenance fluids, smaller cannulae (pink/blue) are fine. In an emergency, a large cannula is preferred (green or bigger) since this permits more rapid administration of medications and fluids

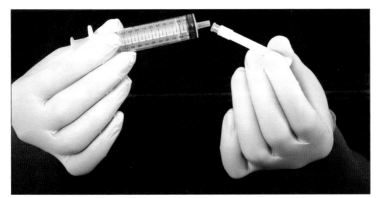

'Patient comfort is very important in considering where to place the cannula, particularly in non emergency situations. Put it in the left arm if they are right handed, use a small cannula if that is all that might be needed, and remember that although the antecubital fossa is tempting, placing a cannula here makes moving the arm more difficult'

Explaining Cannulation to the Patient

1. A cannula is a small plastic tube that remains in your vein allowing you to receive fluid and medication

2. It is inserted using a needle, a bit like having a blood test. You will feel a sharp scratch but the needle is removed once the plastic tube is in place

3. It is held in place with a sticky dressing

4. The cannula will be changed every three days if you need it for a longer period of time

5. It may take a few attempts to ensure the plastic tube is in the correct place

Performing the Procedure

Preparing the Flush

1. Clean hands and put on non sterile gloves

2. Attach the 21-gauge needle to the 10 mL syringe (leave the sheath on for now) (Fig 3.34)

3. Double check that you have selected 0.9% saline, that it is in date, and that the packaging is clean and intact – many IV medications appear in near-identical ampoules

4. Remove the top from the 0.9% saline and draw 10 mL up into your syringe using a 21-gauge needle (Fig 3.35)

5. Expel any air from the syringe by tapping it/advancing the plunger (Fig 3.36)

6. Discard the needle in the sharps bin and attach the syringe to the second needle for storage (or if available, a sterilised cap for the syringe tip)

7. Place the flush into the equipment tray alongside the other cannulation equipment

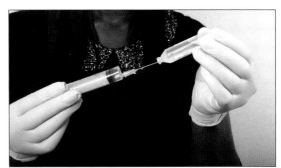

Fig 3.35: Draw up the saline flush

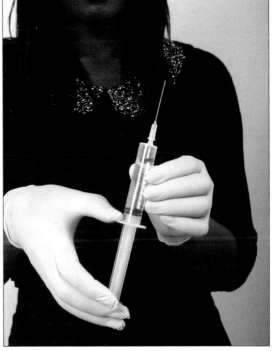

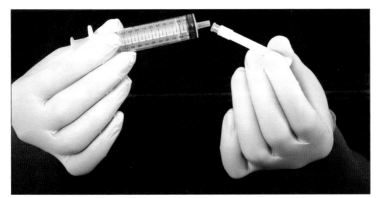

Fig 3.34: Prepare your needle and syringe

Fig 3.36: Expel any air present

Insert the Cannula

1. Remove the cannula from its packaging and open the sterile dressing pack
2. Position the patient's arm comfortably
3. Place the tourniquet approximately 7-10cm proximal to the site of insertion (Fig 3.37)
4. Select vein, then loosen tourniquet
5. Wash hands, put on new non sterile gloves and apron
6. Clean the site using the skin cleansing solution – clean for 30 seconds and leave to air dry (Fig 3.38)
7. Retighten tourniquet
8. Tether the vein that you have selected beneath the insertion site and insert the cannula at approximately 15° using NTT, while warning the patient of a 'sharp scratch' (Fig 3.39)
9. Advance the cannula until flashback is obtained. **Do not repalpate the aseptic area** of the skin at any time during the procedure
10. Once flashback has been seen, advance the cannula slightly further (1-2mm). This ensures the cannula tubing is within the vein before you advance it forward, over and off the needle

'It's fine to re-palpate for a vein, if you've lost it — you just need to clean the skin again, or wear sterile gloves'

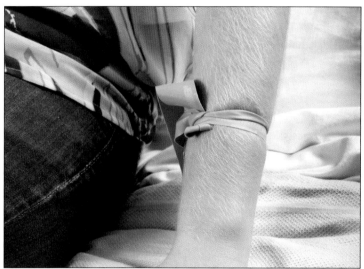

Fig 3.37: Ensure tourniquet out of the sterile field

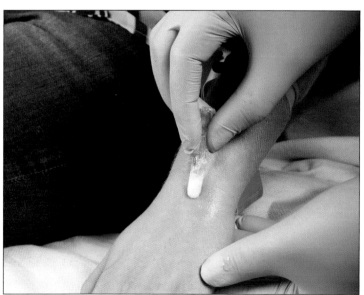

Fig 3.38: Carefully clean cannula insertion site

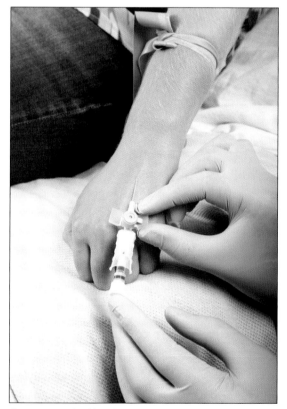

Fig 3.39: Enter the skin using a NTT

11. Hold the needle still and advance the cannula over it, all the way into the vein. No part of the cannula tubing must be seen at the point of entry (Fig 3.40)

12. Release the tourniquet

13. Occlude the vein and cannula with firm pressure (Fig 3.41) and then gently remove the needle

14. Dispose of the needle straight into the sharps bin (Fig 3.42)

15. Depending on Trust policy, attach a cap, bung or IV extension set (which requires separate preparation) on the end of the cannula

16. Wipe away any blood that may have leaked around the cannula with cotton wool

17. Apply sterile adhesive dressing (Fig 3.43)

18. Write the date and time on the cannula dressing label

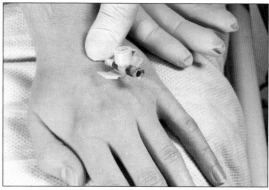
Fig 3.41: Press firmly over the plastic cannula tubing to occlude it

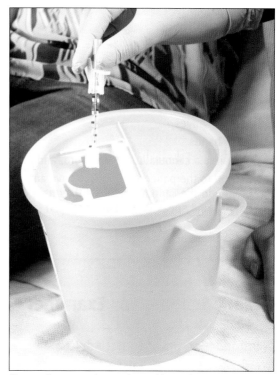
Fig 3.42: Ensure you have a sharps bin nearby

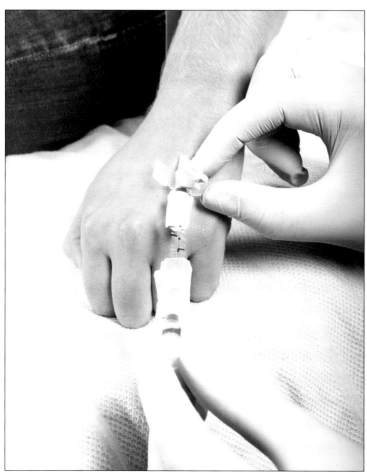
Fig 3.40: Cannula is fully inserted

'As a general rule, if you fail twice at putting a cannula in, ask a senior colleague to place it instead'

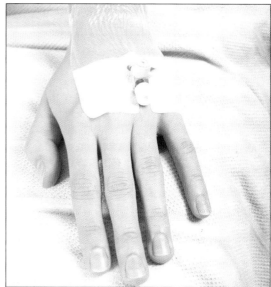
Fig 3.43: Secure the cannula in place

Station 7: SETTING UP A GIVING SET

Mrs Jones has been diagnosed with small bowel obstruction. She has a cannula in situ and now requires maintenance fluid. Please obtain consent for this and then, on the cannulated mannequin provided, demonstrate how to assemble a giving set and commence IV fluid therapy.

Objectives

- To learn how to set up a giving set

General Advice

- Check whether the patient has any concerns or questions and obtain valid consent
- Check if the patient has any allergies
- There are two types of giving sets, one for blood transfusions and another for general use

Equipment Checklist

(remember to check expiry dates on all equipment) (Fig 3.45)

a) IV fluid (e.g. 1L 0.9% saline)
b) Gravity administration set ('Giving Set')
c) Drip stand
d) Skin cleansing solution (e.g. ChloraPrep®)
e) 10 mL syringe
f) 21-gauge needle
g) 10 mL 0.9% saline ampoule for flush
h) Sterile gauze
i) Tray
j) Sharps bin: the sharps bin should always be taken to the point of care
k) 2 x non sterile gloves

Setting up the Giving Set

Preparation

1. Wash hands, put on non-sterile gloves
2. Check the bag of fluid with the examiner:
   - Is it the same fluid and quantity as what is prescribed on the fluid chart?
   - Are any additives required (e.g. potassium or magnesium)?
   - Is it in date?
   - Check that there is no sediment floating in the fluid bag
   - Check that the bag has not leaked into the packaging
3. Remove the bag of fluid from its outer packaging and hang it on the drip stand
4. Remove the giving set from the bag and roll the flow control wheel down to the 'OFF' position. The 'OFF' position is where the tube is clamped, ensuring that the fluid does not run through the line, onto the floor (Fig 3.46)
5. Remove the cap from the fluid bag by twisting it and remove the protective cover from the trocar of the giving set. The trocar is a sharp hollow cylinder that pierces the fluid bag to provide a connection between the fluid and the giving set (take care not to touch either ends in order to maintain an aseptic technique) (Fig 3.47)

Important checks to be made before gathering the necessary equipment include;

- Does the patient have a cannula?
- Is the cannula patent?
- When was the cannula inserted?
- Is there a valid fluid prescription?
- Are any additives to the fluid required?

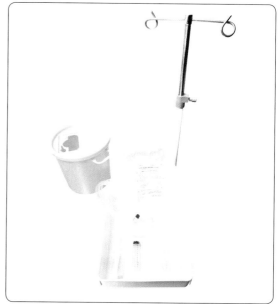

Fig 3.45: Gather the equipment needed

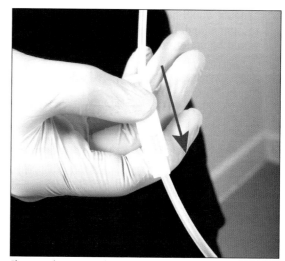

Fig 3.46: Always turn the control wheel to the off position before starting

6. Insert the trocar end of the giving set into the bag of fluid (push hard and twist) (Fig 3.48)

7. Squeeze the chamber at the top of the giving set until it is filled halfway with fluid (Fig 3.49)

8. Slowly open the flow control wheel of the giving set so that fluid flows down the line; do this bit by bit until the line is full of fluid and there are no air bubbles seen; if the line is full of bubbles, the process needs to be started again with new sterile equipment

9. Reset the flow control wheel to the closed position

10. Hang the bag on the drip stand. You are now ready to connect the giving set to the cannula

11. Remove gloves

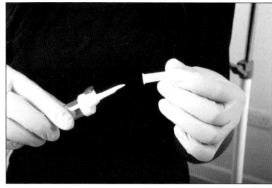

Fig 3.47: Expose the trocar

Connecting the Giving Set to the Cannula

1. Before going to the patient's bedside, draw up a saline flush (as explained in the previous 'cannulation' section) and place this on the equipment tray

2. Wash hands and put on non-sterile gloves

3. Check patient identification

4. Check the cannula (when was it inserted? Are there any signs of localised infection?)

5. Flush the cannula via the coloured cap with the saline (clean cannula entry site first with chlorhexidine wipe)

6. Place the gauze beneath the end of the cannula

7. Depending on your Trust policy, there are different techniques for connecting a giving set. If there is a cannula cap, this must be swiftly removed, wiped with a chlorhexidine wipe and the giving set connected. If your Trust has a connector, this can be cleaned with a chlorhexidine wipe for 30 seconds and then allow 30 seconds for it to dry. After this, the giving set is connected (Fig 3.50)

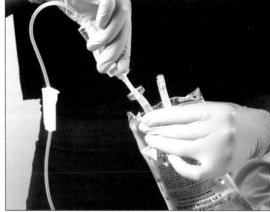

Fig 3.48: Push and twist to insert the trocarr

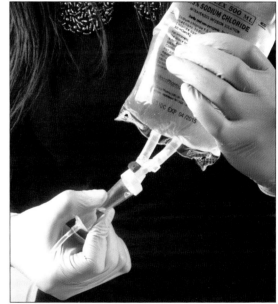

Fig 3.49: Prepare the chamber by squeezing it

Whilst the theory behind IV fluid therapy is complex and beyond the scope of this chapter, it is essential to remember a few key facts when prescribing or administering IV fluids. Broadly speaking, there are two key groups of patients requiring IV fluid;

1. Maintenance – patients with an insufficient oral intake
2. Resuscitation – patients who are hypovolaemic

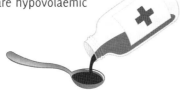

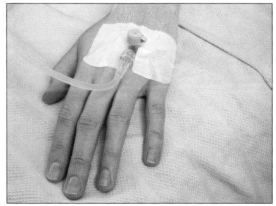

Fig 3.50: Correctly attach the giving set to the cannula

Mark Scheme for Examiner

Introduction and General Advice
Introduces self (clean hands)

Identifies patient (3 points of ID)

Explains procedure, identifies concerns and obtains consent

Checks allergies, checks cannula (insertion date, infection signs), checks fluid prescription

Preparation
Obtains equipment and checks expiry date

Washes hands and puts on non-sterile gloves

Examines fluid bag

Removes the giving set from the bag and closes the flow control wheel

Removes cap from the fluid bag and hangs it on drip stand

Inserts the trocar of the giving set into the bag of fluid

Squeezes the chamber at the top of the giving set until it is filled halfway with fluid

Opens flow control wheel slowly, then closes it when line full of fluid

Ensures IV line is free of air bubbles

Preparation of IV Flush
Draws up saline flush using NTT

Safely stows syringe in tray

Connecting the Giving Set
Washes hands and puts on non-sterile gloves

Cleans end of cannula

Uses appropriate connection technique

Calculating the Drip Rate
Re-checks fluid prescription (for duration of fluid therapy)

Sets flow wheel correctly

Finishing
Disposes of equipment, removes gloves and washes hands

Provides appropriate documentation

General Points
Talks throughout the procedure to the patient and avoids patient contamination

Questions and Answers for Candidate

In an emergency scenario how could you maximise the rate at which you administer IV fluid?

- Insert largest cannula size possible
- Increase drip stand height
- Squeeze fluid bag or apply pressurised cuff
- Insert a second cannula

Additional Questions to Consider

1. What is the difference between crystalloids and colloids and when might you use each?
2. What is a fluid challenge? How would you administer one?
3. What signs would suggest that a patient's cannula is not working correctly?
4. How would you assess the rate at which to give fluid in a dehydrated patient?

Station 8: BLOOD TRANSFUSION

ACUTE PATIENT MANAGEMENT

Mrs Patel is a 72-year-old women who has been admitted to hospital with lethargy, drowsiness and shortness of breath. On examination, she has pale conjunctiva and tachypnoea. Her blood tests have come back demonstrating a normocytic anaemia with an Hb is 65 g/L. Please discuss blood transfusion with the examiner.

Objectives

- Understanding the indications, procedure and complications of blood transfusions

General Advice

- Obtain valid consent
- Each Trust will have a policy for the procedure of administration of blood products. Ensure that you are familiar with these before you start working
- There is no standardised 'trigger' for transfusion
- The decision to transfuse should be taken after considering the laboratory results, the clinical assessment of the patient as well as the risks and benefits of transfusion
- If possible, the decision to transfuse should always be discussed with the patient
- The reason for transfusion must be documented in the patient's notes

Ordering Blood Products

There is a strict process in most Trusts with regards to ordering blood products. Most require the order form to be handwritten and signed by both the healthcare professional that ordered the blood and the person that took the blood. If there is any discrepancy between the order form and the blood sample, the order will not be processed

The labelling of blood samples must be undertaken at the bedside, checking details with the patient and with the patient's ID band

What test can you order?

1. **Group and Save:** the blood bank analyses the samples ABO blood group, Rhesus (D) and common red cell antibodies. This result is then stored on the hospital system
2. **Routine Crossmatch:** the blood bank analyses the samples as for group and save but also screens for any antibodies against compatible blood that is stored in the hospital. This takes approximately 40 minutes
3. **Emergency Crossmatch:** the blood bank analyses the samples ABO blood group only. This takes approximately 10 minutes

Note: Group O negative blood is kept in emergency fridges if there isn't time to wait for an emergency crossmatch

Equipment Checklist

(remember to check expiry dates on all equipment)

a) Tray: either single-use, disposable sterilised tray, or a decontaminated plastic tray that is cleaned pre/post procedure
b) 2 x non-sterile gloves and single use apron
c) Skin cleansing solution
d) Prescribed blood product
e) Prescribed 10 mL 0.9% saline to flush
f) Blood giving set
g) 10 mL syringe
h) 1 x 21-gauge needle
i) Sharps bin

What blood products can you commonly order?

Blood Product	Indications	Shelf-Life
Packed red cells	Acute blood loss	35 days
	Peri-operative transfusion	
	Symptomatic anaemia	
Platelets	Active bleeding caused by platelet dysfunction	5 days
Fresh frozen plasma	Replacing coagulation factor deficiency	1-2 years
	Disseminated intravascular coagulation	
	Massive blood transfusion	
	Warfarin reversal (if major bleeding or emergency surgery)	
Cryoprecipitate	Liver disease with abnormal bleeding	1-2 years
	Disseminated intravascular coagulation	
	Massive blood transfusion	

ACUTE PATIENT MANAGEMENT

Checks and Preparation

1. Check that the patient has given valid consent
2. Wash hands. Put on gloves. Compare the type of blood you have received from the lab with the order form
3. Compare the ABO blood group and Rh(D) reports ensuring they are the same
4. Assess the blood product you have been supplied with, checking for any abnormal colouring, gas bubbles, tampering and expiry date
5. Confirm the patient's identity by checking the identification wristband and asking the patient to state:
   - Full name
   - Date of birth
   - Address and postcode

Confirm with another qualified member of staff (this is stated in some Trust policies)

6. Check that the blood donor number and the patient's number are accurate
7. Document a full set of observations including:
   - Respiratory rate
   - Heart rate
   - Temperature
   - BP
   - SaO$_2$
8. Check that the patient has a patent IV cannula in situ that has been in situ for less than 72 hours
9. Check that the cannula site has no sign of infection
10. Collect the equipment you require and assemble your 0.9% saline flush in a 10 mL syringe
11. Wash hands, don non-sterile gloves and apron
12. Prepare the blood product using a blood giving set (as in station 3.7)

Giving Blood Product

1. Clean the coloured port of the cannula using skin cleansing solution for 30 seconds and allow to dry for 30 seconds
2. Check that the cannula is patent by flushing 5 mL of 0.9% saline through the coloured port of the cannula
3. Once you are sure that the cannula is correctly in place, attach the blood transfusion giving set and start the transfusion (Fig 3.51)
4. Wash hands and remove gloves
5. Remain with the patient for at least 15-30 minutes, depending on Trust guidelines

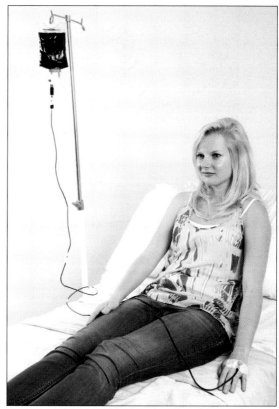

Fig 3.51: Administer the blood product through a cannula

Documenting the Procedure

Document under the following headings:

- Date and time transfusion started
- Date and time transfusion finished
- Reason for transfusion
- Patient consent
- Type of blood product
- Number of units transfused
- Unit numbers
- Outcome of transfusion
- Adverse reactions (if any)

Repeat and document the patient's general observations every 5-10 minutes as recommended by your Trust guidelines

There are numerous transfusion related complications, some of which are highlighted below. An acute reaction is defined as occurring within 24 hours of the transfusion being given, whilst a delayed reaction is defined as one starting after 24 hours

ACUTE

Acute haemolysis	Usually presents with: pyrexia, pain, tachycardia, hypotension and agitation
Anaphylaxis	Usually presents with: wheeze, flushing, tachypnoea, tachycardia and hypotension
Febrile non-haemolytic transfusion reaction	Usually presents with: isolated pyrexia
Transfusion related circulatory overload	Usually presents with: hypertension, tachypnoea and tachycardia

DELAYED

Viral infection	These include: hepatitis B and hepatitis C
Delayed haemolytic reaction	As for acute haemolysis

Guidelines:

UK Blood Transfusion and Tissue Transplantation Services http://www.transfusionguidelines.org.uk/index.aspx

British Committee for Standards in Haematology http://www.bcshguidelines.com/

Mark Scheme for Examiner

Introduction and General Advice

Introduces self (clean hands)

Identifies patient (3 points of ID) and confirms with another staff member

Explains procedure, identifies concerns and obtains consent

Preparation

Obtains equipment, checks expiry dates, washes hands, dons gloves

Assembles equipment

Checks prescription

Checks blood product and confirms with another staff member

Documents full set of patient observations

Checks cannula site

Washes hands, dons non-sterile gloves and apron

Giving Blood Product

Cleans cannula port and draws up saline flush

Checks cannula patency

Sets up blood transfusion giving set

Starts transfusion

Washes hands, removes gloves and apron

Remains with patient

Repeats and documents observations

Disposes of equipment and cleans tray

Documentation

Date and time transfusion started

Date and time transfusion finished

Reason for transfusion

Patient consent

Type of blood product

Number of units transfused

Unit numbers

Outcome of transfusion

Adverse reactions (if any)

General Points

Talks throughout the procedure to the patient

Avoids patient contamination, i.e. NTT

Questions and Answers for Candidate

How do you know how many units to transfuse?

- This depends on the individual situation of the patient you are caring for. If you are unsure it is best to ask the advice of a senior doctor on your team, or the duty Haematologist. As a general rule, 1 unit of packed red cells will increase the Hb by approximately 10g/L

When do you decide to transfuse?

- This depends on the individual situation of the patient you are caring for. If you are unsure it is best to ask for advice. As a general rule, guidelines tend to recommend transfusing when a patient's Hb falls below 70-80g/L; however, if a patient has co-morbidities such as ischaemic heart disease, this threshold may be increased to 100g/L. Lower transfusion threshold are also considered in patients symptomatic of anaemia

When would you consider giving a blood transfusion at night?

- Most Trusts recommend transfusing a patient during the day as there are more staff present on the wards and it is safer for the patient, as these patients require regular observations during and after transfusion. There are specific areas in the hospital and certain situations when a transfusion will be given overnight, for example ITU, A&E and the medical or surgical assessment units. However, blood transfusions can be given anytime in an emergency

Additional Questions to Consider

1. What is the difference between a blood giving set and a regular giving set?

2. What other treatments can be used instead of a blood transfusion for anaemic patients?

3. Over what length of time should a unit of red cell concentrate be given?

4. When would you consider giving diuretics with a blood transfusion?

5. What are the causes of a normocytic anaemia?

ACUTE PATIENT MANAGEMENT

Station 9: ECGs

Mr Edmonds has come to the Emergency Department with central crushing chest pain. He has hypertension and is a smoker. An ECG has been performed. Please interpret it and present your findings.

Objectives of the Station

- To learn how to perform an ECG
- To learn how to interpret an ECG
- To learn management of common ECG findings

Performing an ECG

There is a universal standard when performing a 12-lead ECG. There are six chest leads and four limb leads that are attached to the patient.

The chest leads are labelled V1-V6 and are positioned as following: (Fig 3.52)

- V1: 4th intercostal space, right sternal edge
- V2: 4th intercostal space, left sternal edge
- V3: site midway between V2 and V4
- V4: 5th intercostal space, mid-clavicular line
- V5: 5th intercostal space, anterior axillary line
- V6: 5th intercostal space, mid-axillary line

The limb leads are positioned as following: (Fig 3.53)

- aVR: right wrist/shoulder (**red lead**)
- aVL: left wrist/shoulder (yellow lead)
- aVF: left ankle (green lead)
- N: right ankle (**black lead**)

These leads are attached and generate a 12-lead ECG recording

General Advice

- Obtain valid consent
- Remove any body hair over areas that you wish to attach the ECG leads to
- Ensure the patient is lying on a bed, or sitting comfortably, and still
- Adequately expose the patient. This may involve bra removal in female patients
- Inform female patients that the chest electrode stickers will be placed underneath their breast
- Ask the patient if they have any allergies. Patients may be allergic to the electrode sticker adhesive

Recording the ECG

1. Check the machine's calibration with the 1mV signal (normally 1cm =1mV)
2. Set the recording speed to 25mm/s
3. Wash your hands
4. Place 10 electrode stickers on the patient's skin in the correct positions outlined above
5. Ensures the electrode stickers are placed with the small tab downwards. This ensures the lead clips will lie flat against the patients skin
6. Attach the electrodes to the stickers

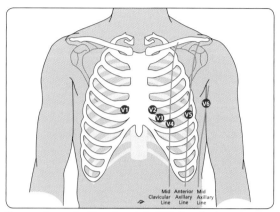

Fig 3.52: Anatomical location of the ECG chest leads

7. Check that all the electrode stickers and electrodes are correctly attached to the patient
8. Ask the patient to remain still and quiet
9. Press the 'RECORD' button
10. Check the printed ECG to ensure that there is a good trace
11. Repeat the ECG if there is a poor trace

Finishing

1. Label the ECG with the patients details
2. Remove the electrodes and the electrode stickers from the patient
3. Ask the patient to get dressed and offer assistance if required
4. Document the ECG recording in the notes and interpret it

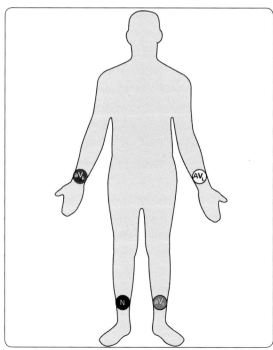

Fig 3.53: Anatomical position of ECG limb leads

Now we will discuss how to interpret an ECG recording

Important information to note when reporting an ECG:

- Time and date of ECG
- Patient details (name, date of birth)
- Calibration
- Paper speed – usually 25 mm/second (one small square = 40 msec)
- Heart rate
- Heart rhythm
- Cardiac axis
- Morphology

ECG changes in Hyperkalaemia

- Tall tented T waves
- Flattened P waves and prolonged PR interval
- Widened QRS complexes which can merge with the T wave to produce a sine wave pattern

Heart Rate

First assess if the heart rhythm is regular or irregular.

- If regular, count the number of large boxes between adjacent R waves
  o   Divide this number by 300
  o   For example, if there are 3 large boxes between R waves, 300/3 = a heart rate of 100 beats per minute
- If irregular, the heart rate may still be roughly estimated. The rhythm strip normally corresponds to 10 seconds of electrical activity. The number of R waves present in the rhythm strip can therefore by multiplied by six to give the number of heart beats each minute

  For example, if there were 22 RR intervals on the 10 second rhythm strip, the heart rate is 22 x 6 = 132 beats per minute (alternatively, dividing the number of large squares between 3 RR intervals into 900 is another way to calculate irregular rates)

Normal heart rate is defined as 60-100 beats per minute. A HR >100 is defined as a tachycardia; a HR <60 is defined as bradycardia. Note that not all tachycardias and bradycardias are pathological and often reflect the physiologic state, e.g. sleeping, exercising and stress

Tachycardia

Broad complex tacharrhythmia

- Ventricular tachycardia (Fig 3.54)
- Torsades de Pointes (Fig 3.55)

Management:

Such rhythms of broad complex tachyarrhythmia are potentially life threatening and should be managed immediately;

- Resuscitate using an ABC approach
- Oxygen
- Put out crash call
- Obtain IV access
- Identify reversible causes such as electrolyte imbalances
- The decision to administer DC shock or medication will depend on the haemodynamic status of the patient as well as the type of rhythm identified. Note: Supraventricular tachycardia with aberrant conduction can look like ventricular tachycardia. If in doubt, treat as ventricular tachycardia

ACUTE PATIENT MANAGEMENT

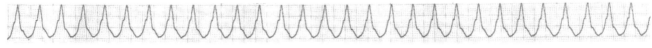

Fig 3.54: Ventricular Tachycardia (regular rhythm, with broad complexes)

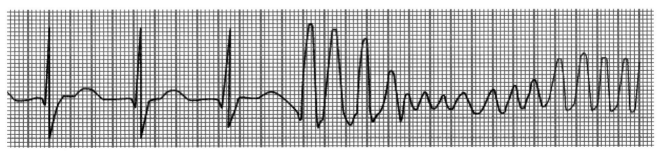

Fig 3.55: Torsades de Pointes (evolves on the right of this ECG strip- note the height of the complexes gradually decreases and then increases)

Continues overleaf...

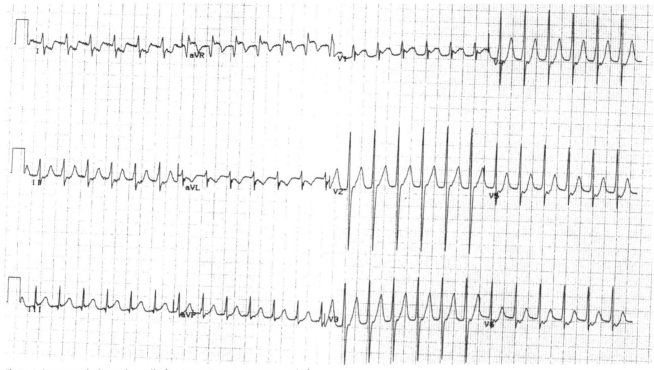

Fig 3.56: Supraventricular tachycardia (no P waves seen, narrow complex)

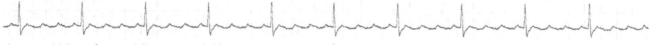

Fig 3.57: Atrial flutter (saw tooth flutter waves visable, narrow complex, regular)

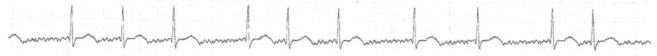

Fig 3.58: Atrial fibrillation (no P waves, narrow complex, irregularly irregular)

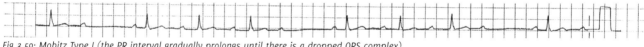

Fig 3.59: Mobitz Type I (the PR interval gradually prolongs until there is a dropped QRS complex)

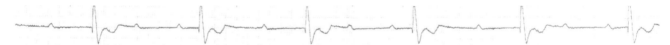

Fig 3.60: 3rd degree heart block (complete dissociation between P waves and QRS complexes)

Narrow Complex Tachycardia

- Supraventricular tachycardia (Fig 3.56)
- Atrial flutter (Fig 3.57)
- Atrial fibrillation with fast ventricular response (Fig 3.58)

Management

- Resuscitate using an ABC approach
- If haemodynamically unstable, put out a crash call as the patient my require DC cardioversion
- Inform a senior if the patient is stable and doesn't require a crash team
- If the rhythm is regular, try vagal maneuver
  - o Ask patient to perform a vagal maneuver by asking them to blow into a syringe
  - o Carotid sinus massage
- Consider IV adenosine (6mg IV using cardiac monitoring with full arrest facilities available in case required)
- If the rhythm is irregularly irregular (atrial fibrillation), a beta blocker or digoxin can be used

Bradycardia

- First degree heart block. The PR interval is prolonged but there are no dropped beats
- Second degree heart block Mobitz Type I. The PR interval gradually prolongs until there is a P wave that is not followed by a QRS complex (Fig 3.59)
- Second degree heart block Mobitz Type II. The PR interval is the same but a QRS is dropped in a regular manner
- Complete (third degree) heart block. The P waves and QRS complexes are completely disassociated (Fig 3.60)

Management

- Resuscitate using an ABC approach
- If the patient is haemodynamically stable, then there may be no need to do anything in the acute setting. Identify any medications that may be causing bradycardia, such as beta blockers and arrange for the patient to be on a cardiac monitor if one is available

- If the patient is unstable, inform a senior or put out a crash call
- 500 micrograms of atropine should be considered
- The patient may need transcutaneous or internal pacing as a temporary measure

Cardiac Axis

- The cardiac axis is the overall direction of the wave of ventricular depolarisation (measured in the vertical plane)
- This is measured from a zero reference point (from the same viewpoint as Lead I)
- An axis above this line is denoted by a negative number (of degrees) and an axis lying below this line is given a positive number (of degrees)

Axis	Lead I	Lead AVF
Normal	+	+
Left Axis Deviation*	+	-
Right Axis Deviation	-	+
Extreme Right Axis Deviation	-	-

There are several ways to calculate the axis. Here is the simplest: A lead is 'positive' if there is a greater positive deflection in the QRS complex than the negative deflection (i.e. the R wave is taller than the S wave). A negative lead has a greater negative deflection.

*Note this table is a simplification. The most accurate method of determining the axis is to work out the exact angle of the axis. Remember also that a negative aVF, with a positive lead 1, can be normal if it is in the zero to -30 degree range. However, most doctors use this simplification in everyday practice

Wave Morphology

P Waves

- If all the P waves in the rhythm strip are of similar morphology, it is likely that they are arising from the same focus
- If tall: consider right atrium enlargement ('P pulmonale')
- If bifid: consider left atrium enlargement ('P mitrale')
- If flattened: consider hyperkalemia

QRS Complex

If widened (>120ms), there is a bundle branch block present. Using the mnemonic 'WILLIAM MARROW' can be helpful

- WiLLiaM (L for left bundle branch block – WM corresponds to V1 looking like 'W' and V6 looking like 'M'. There are deep S wave in leads V1-3, and tall R waves in V5-6) (Fig 3.61)
- MaRRoW (R for right bundle branch block – MW corresponds to V1 looking like 'M' and V6 looking like 'W' There is a second R wave in V1-3 and a wide slurred S wave in lead V5-6) (Fig 3.62)
- New onset left bundle branch block in the setting of suspected acute coronary syndrome should be managed the same as ST elevation myocardial infarction (STEMI)

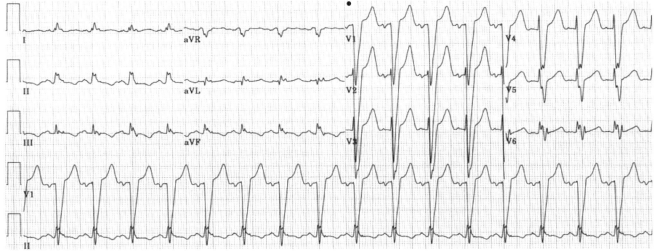

Fig 3.61: Left bundle branch block

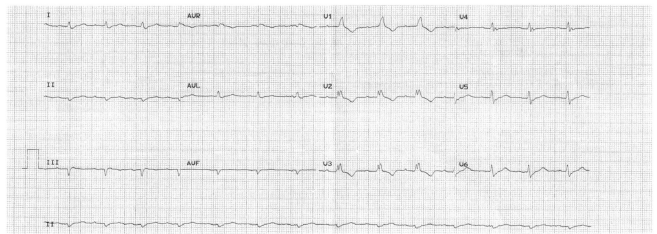

Fig 3.62: Right bundle branch block

Causes of right bundle branch block

Normal variant

Myocardial infarction

Pulmonary embolism

Cor pulmonale

Congenital heart disease

Cardiomyopathy

Causes of left bundle branch block

Myocardial infarction

Hypertension

Conduction system fibrosis

Cardiomyopathy

ST Segments

The important changes to look for are either elevation or depression. The two important differentials for ST elevation are pericarditis and myocardial infarction (MI)

NOTE: in the presence of left bundle branch block, the ST segments cannot be accurately interpreted

	ST Elevation MI	**Pericarditis**
Site	ST elevation localised to ischemic territory	Widespread 'saddle-shaped' ST elevation
ST Depression	Reciprocal ST depression e.g. ST depression in the anterior territory with an inferior infarct	No reciprocal change
PR Segment	Normal	PR depression

Other causes of ST elevation include left ventricular aneurysm. ST elevation may also be confused with early repolarisation

Causes of ST depression include:
- Myocardial ischaemia
- Digoxin ('reverse tick' appearance of ST segment)
- Left/right ventricular hypertrophy
- Bundle branch block
- Hypokalaemia

Q Wave Changes

A pathological Q waves is one which is greater than 1/3rd of the height of the R wave on the same QRS complex and has a duration of greater than 40 ms. This is suggestive of an old infarct

In the context of an evolving infarct, if Q waves develop on serial ECGs, this is suggestive of a completed infarct

T Wave Changes

The two most important causes of T wave change are myocardial ischemia and hyperkalaemia

Ischemic T Wave changes:
- T wave inversion (can be normal in V1, III and aVR, especially if present in old ECGs)
- Flattened T waves
- Biphasic T waves
- Peaked T waves

If T wave inversion occurs across several leads, in the same myocardial territory, myocardial ischaemia becomes more likely

Hyperkalemia is associated will tall tented T waves

Ischaemic changes on ECG

STEMI

- Corresponds to total coronary artery occlusion
- ST elevation will be in the leads that correspond to a particular territory of a coronary artery
- ST segments are considered to be elevated if > 1mm in limb leads and > 1mm in chest leads
- An important differential for ST elevation is pericarditis. ST elevation in pericarditis is often in all the leads and is saddle shaped
- Dominant R waves in lead V1-3, with significant ST depression is suggestive of a posterior STEMI which is easily missed if not actively looked for

Management of STEMI

- Resuscitate using an ABC approach
- Oxygen to maintain SaO$_2$ 95-98%
- Aspirin (300 mg)
- Sublingual GTN (1-2 puffs) and clopidogrel (300mg)
- IV morphine (1-10 mg titrated to pain)
- If available, contact the cardiology emergency team with a view to arranging Primary Coronary Intervention
- Once stable, the priority is to restore coronary perfusion as soon as possible
- It is helpful to take a full set of bloods including a troponin and clotting

'Always try and compare a new ECG to an old one so that acute changes are more obvious and chronic abnormalities aren't taken as new changes. It can sometimes be difficult to differentiate between true ST segment elevation and 'high take off' of the ST segment into the T wave. It is always important to correlate the ECG with the patient's symptoms and if in doubt, seek a second opinion from a senior colleague'

- T wave inversion and/or ST depression
- Indicates subtotal occlusion of coronary artery
- NSTEMI can only be diagnosed with the presence of a raised troponin

Management of NSTEMI

- Resuscitate using an ABC approach
- Oxygen to maintain SaO_2 95-98%
- Sublingual GTN (1-2 puffs)
- Aspirin (300 mg)
- Clopidogrel (300 mg)
- Low molecular weight heparin or factor Xa inhibitor e.g. Fondaparinux (2.5 mg)
- IV morphine (1-10 mg titrated to pain)
- Blood tests including troponin and clotting
- Inform a senior
- Serial ECGs

Note: The management of MIs may vary between trusts. Ensure you are familiar with the protocols of the trust you are working in

Anatomical Relations of ECG Leads

- II, III, aVF: inferior surface (right coronary artery or left circumflex)
- V1, V2, V3, V4: anterior surface (left anterior descending coronary artery)
- I, aVL, V5, V6: lateral surface (left coronary artery, circumflex)
- V5, V6: high lateral leads (left coronary artery, circumflex)

Rhythm

1. Are normal P waves present?
2. Is each P wave followed by a QRS complex?

If yes to both of the above questions, the rhythm is sinus

3. What is the PR interval? (i.e. looking for heart block)
   o If there are P waves, is the PR interval the same for each QRS complex?
   o Is the PR interval the normal length (3-5 small squares (120 - 200 ms))?
4. What is the QRS duration?
   o If QRS duration > 120 ms ('broad complex'), the focus of an arrhythmia will usually be coming from within the ventricles, e.g. ventricular tachycardia. If there is a P wave preceding each QRS, it would indicate aberrant conduction due to LBBB, RBBB or ventricular pre-excitation due to Wolff-Parkinson-White syndrome, but the PR interval is short in Wolff-Parkinson White syndrome
   o A QRS duration < 120 ms ('narrow complex') implies ventricular depolarisation via the His / Purkinjie system, which can only occur with a supra-ventricular focus

Putting it all together – reporting an ECG

- Remember the report has two parts – describing the ECG and interpretation of it
- Follow the same order for each ECG you report:
  o Patient details, date and time of ECG
  o Rate
  o Rhythm
  o Axis
  o P waves and PR interval
  o QRS complexes
    - Duration
    - Presence of Q waves
    - Height of R and S waves
  o ST segments
  o T waves

Vessels

- Trace the 4 major vessel arcs out to the periphery
- Veins appear darker than arteries

Look for:

- o Arteriovenous (AV) nipping (at vessel crossing points), e.g. hypertension
- o Haemorrhages or vessel tortuosity, e.g. diabetes/hypertension
- o Microaneurysms, e.g. diabetes
- o Silver wiring, e.g. hypertension

Periphery

- Examine each quadrant, ensuring that the retina looks pink and healthy
- Due to the magnification of the ophthalmoscope, it is difficult to visualise the periphery

Diabetic Retinopathy

- The main risk factor for diabetic retinopathy is the length of time the person has had diabetes
- All patients with diabetes should be screened for retinopathy at least annually
- Incidence is lower with excellent glycaemic control

Non-Proliferative Diabetic Retinopathy (NPDR) (Fig 3.65)

- Microaneurysms (smaller, and more distinct than dot haemorrhage, but difficult to differentiate the two)
- 'Dot and blot' haemorrhages
- Hard exudates
- Cotton wool spots (due to local ischaemia)
- Normal visual acuity
- No treatment indicated, only regular follow-up

Severe Non-Proliferative Diabetic

- Venous beading/dilatation/tortuosity
- Larger and more widespread blot haemorrhages
- Intraretinal microvascular abnormality
- Closer follow-up

Proliferative Diabetic Retinopathy

- Neovascularisation (due to ischaemia): new vessels on the disc/elsewhere
- Risk of vitreous haemorrhage (new vessels are friable and prone to bleeding, particularly those close to the disc)
- Risk of tractional retinal detachment
- Severe loss of vision may occur secondary to these, neovascularisation is an indication for urgent referral for photocoagulation

Diabetic Maculopathy

- Vessel leakage and/or ischemia at the macula
- Most common cause of visual loss in diabetes

Common Causes of Visual Loss

Acute	Gradual
Uveitis	Cataract
Keratitis, e.g. due to corneal ulcer	Age-related macular degeneration
Optic neuritis	Optic neuropathy (including glaucoma)
Ischaemic optic neuropathy	
Retinal vein/artery occlusion	
Retinal detachment	
Vitreous haemorrhage	
Stroke	

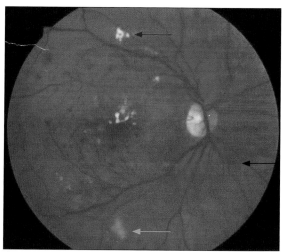

Fig 3.65: Features of NPDR; dot and blot haemorrhages (black arrow), hard exudates (blue arrow) and cotton wool spots (green arrow)

Laser Treatment Scars

- Panretinal photocoagulation (PRP) is used for proliferative diabetic retinopathy
- Focal/grid laser photocoagulation is used for diabetic maculopathy

Hypertensive Retinopathy (Fig 3.66)

- Arteriolar narrowing
- Arterio-venous nipping at crossing points
- Copper/silver wiring (increased central light reflex from arterioles)
- Cotton wool spots
- Hard exudates, which may surround the macula forming a partial or complete 'star'
- Blot or flame haemorrhages
- Usually asymptomatic if chronic

Accelerated Hypertension

- Disc swelling, indicating an optic neuropathy, as well as retinopathy changes above
- May have reduced visual acuity
- Usually severe hypertension (e.g. systolic BP >220mmHg) and evidence of other end-organ damage

Papilloedema (Fig 3.67)

- Bilateral disc swelling secondary to raised intracranial pressure
- Blurred disc margins ± disc pallor
- If long-standing, you may see dilated veins and hard exudates

Optic Neuritis

- Inflammation or demyelination

Anterior Ischaemic Optic Neuropathy

- Infarction of the optic nerve head, usually secondary to giant cell arteritis or hypertension

Age-related Macular Degeneration (AMD)

- Commonest cause of blindness in the developed world for over 50s

Dry (atrophic) AMD (Fig 3.68)

- Degeneration at and around the macula. More common than wet AMD
- Atrophic (pale) +/- hyperpigmented areas
- Drusen (subretinal deposits of waste products)
- No treatment

Wet (neovascular) AMD

- Choroidal neovascularisation, which may leak, leading to oedema and haemorrhage
- More rapid loss of vision
- Anti-VEGF injections into the vitreous or sometimes laser treatment may be given

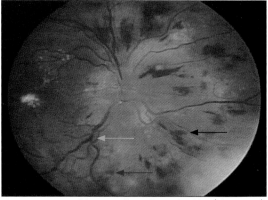

Fig 3.66 Features of hypertensive retinopathy; blot (blue arrow) and flame-shaped haemorrhages (black arrow), arterio-venous nipping (green arrow)

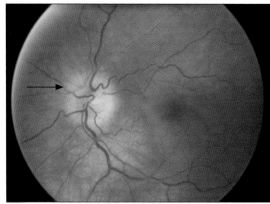

Fig 3.67: Features of papilloedema; blurred margins (black arrow, which indicates a swollen optic disc)

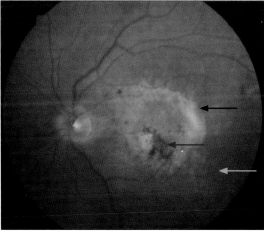

Fig 3.68: Features of dry AMD; pale area around the macula (black arrow), hyperpigmented areas (blue arrow) and soft drusen (green arrow)

ACUTE PATIENT MANAGEMENT

Mark Scheme for Examiner

Introduction and General Preparation

Introduces self (washes hands)

Identifies patient (3 points of ID)

Explains procedure and obtains consent

Warns the patient about the need to be close to their face

Positioning and Technique

Darkens room and patient asked to sit

Dilates pupils if needed

Correct technique and adjustment of ophthalmoscope

Uses correct hand to hold ophthalmoscope when examining

Examination

Elicits the red reflex

Examines the optic disc

Examines the macula

Examines the peripheries in all four quadrants

Reports findings appropriately

Explains findings to patient

Questions and Answers for Candidate

What are the differential diagnoses of a 'red eye'?

* Subconjunctival haemorrhage
* Conjunctivitis
* Glaucoma
* Anterior uveitis
* Scleritis/Episcleritis

What are some causes of a relative afferent pupil defect (RAPD)?

* Optic neuritis
* Optic atrophy
* Papillitis
* Retinal detachments
* Central retinal artery occlusion
* Widespread retinal disease
* Optic nerve compression

Additional Questions to Consider

1. How can you tell the difference between a stye and a chalazion?
2. What would you see in a third nerve palsy?
3. How does blepharitis present?
4. What is the difference between scleritis and episcleritis?
5. How is a dendritic ulcer classically visualised and what does it look like?

Station 11: OTOSCOPY

Mr Downing is an 82-year-old man complaining of difficulty hearing the television over the last few months. Perform an otoscopic examination to evaluate the cause of his hearing loss.

Objectives

- To learn how to perform otoscopy
- To learn how to interpret common findings on otoscopy

Equipment

- Clean disposable speculum (one for each ear)
- Otoscope

Examination

1. Select a 4mm speculum and attach it to the otoscope
2. Turn the otoscope to full brightness
3. Hold the otoscope and place your little finger on the patients zygoma to ensure you have full control of the otoscope at all times
4. Lift the pinna upwards and backwards with your other hand (Fig 3.69)
5. Place the speculum on the posterior aspect of the tragus and then carefully insert the speculum into the ear canal whilst looking through the otoscope
   - Examine the external auditory meatus
   - Take note of any evidence of infection or wax build up within the ear canal
   - Try to identify the different parts of the tympanic membrane and make note of any abnormalities seen
6. Repeat the examination with the other ear

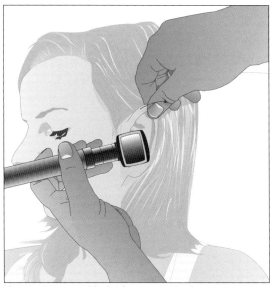

Fig 3.69: Correct positioning for ear examination

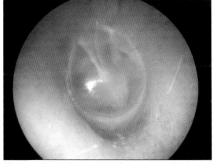

Fig 3.70: Normal anatomy of the tympanic membrane

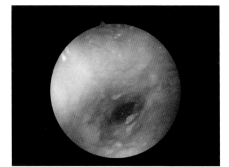

Fig 3.71: Acute otitis externa

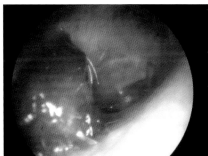

Fig 3.72: Ear wax within ear canal

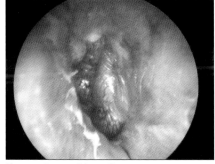

Fig 3.73: Acute otitis media

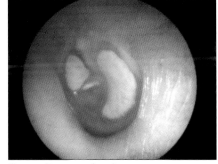

Fig 3.74: Tympanosclerosis

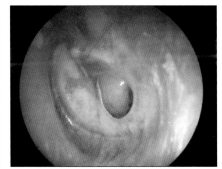

Fig 3.75: Perforated tympanic membrane

Present Your Findings

Mr Downing is an 82-year-old man presenting with progressive hearing loss over the past three months. On otoscopic examination, there is hard brownish yellow cerumen (ear wax) that obscures the tympanic membrane and appears to be impacted on both sides. This is most likely to be the cause of Mr Downing's hearing loss but I would like to complete my examination by performing Rinne's and Weber's tests and reassess Mr Downing's hearing once the ear wax has been removed.

Mark Scheme for Examiner

Introduction and General Preparation

Introduces self (washes hands)

Identifies patient (3 points of ID)

Explains procedure and obtains consent

Warns the patient about the need to place a speculum within the ear canal

Positioning and Technique

Stabilises hand by resting the little finger on the patients zygoma

Carefully places the speculum onto the tragus and then into the ear canal

Examination

Examines the ear canal and describes any abnormalities present

Examines the tympanic membrane and describes any abnormalities present

Uses a clean speculum for examination of the other ear

Reports findings appropriately

Explains findings to patient

Questions and Answers for Candidate

What factors predispose someone to the development of acute otitis externa?

- Absence of ear wax
- High humidity
- Water in the ear canal
- Trauma due to cotton swabs or hearing aids

What are the indications for the removal of ear wax?

- Total occlusion of the ear canal causing hearing loss, earache or tinnitus
- When direct visualisation of the tympanic membrane is required for diagnostic purposes
- In order to take an impression of the ear canal for a hearing aid mould, or if wax is causing the aid to whistle

What are the complications of otitis media?

- Glue ear
- Perforated tympanic membrane
- Mastoiditis (which can lead to meningitis)

Additional Questions to Consider

1. What is tympanosclerosis and how is it treated?
2. What can be done to prevent recurrent ear infections?
3. What is a cholesteatoma and how does it present?
4. At what point should a hearing aid be considered in the elderly?
5. What are the different types of hearing loss and how do they differ?

Station 12: CENTRAL VENOUS LINES

Mr Arnold is a 30-year-old man with known chronic liver disease who has presented acutely with haematemesis. He is a known IV drug user. As the junior doctor on call, you are asked to see him and, after determining he is physiologically stable, you attempt to cannulate him in order to obtain blood samples and to administer IV fluids. Whilst you struggle to find a peripheral vein suitable for cannulation, Mr Arnold vomits a large volume of fresh blood and becomes haemodynamically unstable. You call for help, and after further attempts at peripheral venous access fail, your registrar prepares to insert a central line. Discuss with the examiner the indications for this procedure, key aspects of insertion and how this procedure might guide fluid resuscitation.

Objectives

- Be able to recall the indications for central venous cannulation
- Know the general principles of insertion technique
- Be familiar with the concept of central venous pressure (CVP) monitoring

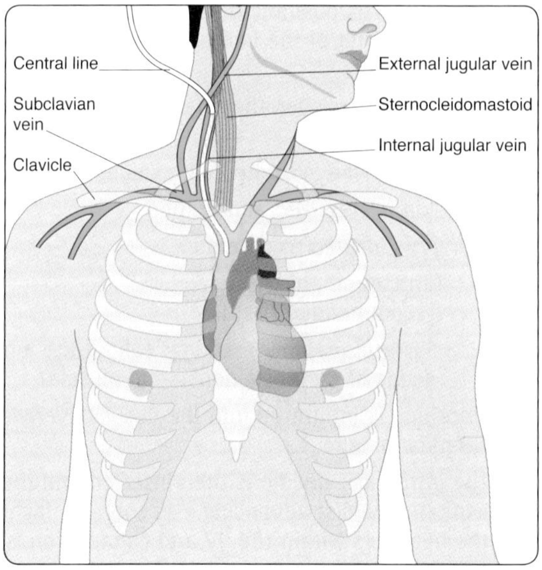

General Advice

- Inserting a central venous catheter (or 'central line') is a complex procedure and as such you would not be expected to perform it as a junior doctor without instruction from an experienced senior colleague
- Central venous cannulation involves the insertion of a catheter into the internal jugular vein or subclavian vein (see 3.76)
- There are several indications for central venous cannulation;
  - o Poor peripheral venous access
  - o CVP monitoring
  - o Total parenteral nutrition infusion
  - o Inotropic or vasoactive drug infusion
  - o Chemotherapy
  - o Haemodialysis
- There are numerous different types of central venous catheter, categories of which include;
  - o Tunnelled and non-tunnelled (tunnelled for more long-term use)
  - o Implantable ports
  - o Peripherally inserted central catheters (PICC)
  - o Dialysis catheters (VASCATH)
- These, in turn, may be single-lumen or multi-lumen catheters, depending on the intended use of the central line (e.g. a multi-lumen catheter would allow several drugs to be infused and CVP to be monitored simultaneously)

Fig 3.76: Anatomical diagram of the major vessels involved in central line insertion

Equipment Checklist

(Remember to check expiry dates on all equipment) (Fig 3.77)

a) Procedure trolley with sterile drape and swabs. Sharps bin
b) Sterile gown
c) Sterile gloves
d) Skin cleansing solution (e.g. chlorhexidine)
e) 10 mL syringe
f) 25-gauge and 21-gauge needles
g) 10 mL 1% lidocaine
h) Seldinger central venous line pack
i) Ultrasound machine
j) Suture and suturing equipment
k) 0.9% saline (for priming and flushing central line)
l) Sterile dressing
m) Scalpel

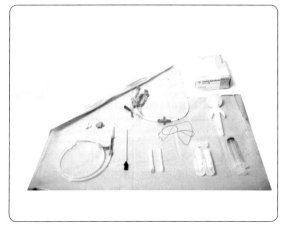

Fig 3.77: Ensure you have all the equipment you require before heading to the bedside

Equipment Checklist

(remember to check expiry dates on all equipment)

a) Tray: either single-use, disposable sterilised tray, or a decontaminated plastic tray that is cleaned pre/post procedure
b) Non-sterile gloves
c) Skin cleansing solution
d) 21-25-gauge needle(s)
e) 21-gauge needle or filter needle for drawing up medication
f) Medication for injection
g) Syringe (size depending on injection)
h) Sharps bin: the sharps bin should always be taken to the point of care

Note: Skin cleansing solutions and method will vary depending on local policy

Preparation for all Injections

1. Obtain consent
2. Wash hands and don a pair of non-sterile gloves
3. Inspect the proposed site for injection and ensure it is suitable
4. Clean site following local policy. Allow to dry fully
5. With a colleague, check the drug dose against the drug chart and check the drug expiry date
6. Draw up the medication using a syringe and a 21-gauge needle if using a plastic ampoule, or a filter needle if using a glass ampoule
7. Expel any excess air in the syringe

LA Injection

1. Discard the 21-gauge needle in the sharps bin and replace with a new 25-gauge needle
2. Hold the syringe like a pencil between your thumb and forefinger
3. Insert the needle at 10-15° into the taut injection site and slowly infiltrate until you see bleb formation (Fig 4.11)
4. Then, if required, change the 25-gauge needle to a 21-gauge needle for deeper infiltration, insert the needle at 45° or 90° through the anaesthetised skin and draw back in the syringe for 5 seconds to check that the needle has not penetrated a vein (Fig 4.12)
5. If there is no flashback, then proceed. If there is flashback, withdraw the needle slightly and re-check for flashback
6. Slowly infiltrate the anaesthetic at a rate in accordance with the instructions. The depth and amount of LA given will depend on the specific procedure
7. Remove the needle carefully and immediately dispose of it in the sharps bin
8. Wait a few minutes before starting the procedure and always check that the skin is anaesthetised before beginning
9. At the end of the procedure, inform the patient to let a member of staff know if the site is painful, bleeds, or if they have any other concerns
10. Remove gloves and wash hands
11. Document the drug administration in the drug chart

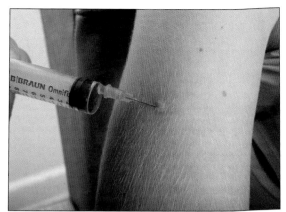
Fig 4.11: A bleb of LA should be seen under the skin

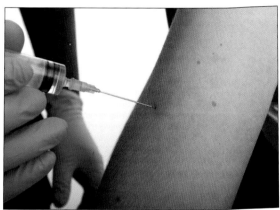
Fig 4.12: If required, reposition the needle for deeper infiltration

Examples of the different LAs used are:
- 1% Lidocaine
- Levobupivacaine
- Prilocaine

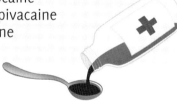

Mark Scheme for Examiner

Introduction and General Advice

Introduces self (clean hands)

Identifies patient (3 points of ID)

Explains procedure, identifies concerns and obtains consent

Checks for allergies and needle phobia

Preparation

Obtains equipment and checks expiry dates

Washes hands, dons non-sterile gloves

Attaches syringe to needle for drawing up medication

Selects appropriate site for injection

Cleans injection site

Checks medication and prescription with colleague

Draws up medication

LA Injection

Checks for flashback before injecting

Begins with intradermal bleb at 15° under the skin and checks response

Administers appropriate amount of LA at 90° or 45°
and to the correct depth for the specific procedure

Waits for the LA to take effect before continuing with specific procedure

Disposes of sharps

Finishing

Tells patient to inform staff if site becomes painful or continues to bleed

Signs the patient's drug chart

Disposes of equipment and cleans tray

Removes gloves and washes hands

General Points

Talks throughout the procedure to the patient

Avoids patient contamination (i.e. NTT)

MEDICATION ADMINISTRATION

Questions and Answers for Candidate

Why is local anaesthetic sometimes used with adrenaline?

- The adrenaline stops the LA from being rapidly redistributed by the circulation and therefore its action is enhanced at the required area. Adrenaline must be used with caution in the extremeties due to the potential risk for ischaemia

When might a local anaesthetic injection be needed?

- Suturing
- Wound cleaning
- Minor and major surgery (cataracts, post laparoscopic surgery)
- Topical preparation for cannulation, LP etc.

Additional Questions to Consider

1. What is the duration of action of lidocaine and levobupivacaine?
2. What does performing a 'field block' mean?
3. What is LA toxicity and when does it normally occur?
4. What are the contraindications for using a LA?

Station 5: INTRAVENOUS DRUGS

You are the junior doctor on the ward. One of your post-operative patients, Mrs Chi, has become unwell overnight spiking temperatures and requires IV antibiotics. Please discuss how you would give the antibiotics with your examiner.

MEDICATION ADMINISTRATION

Objectives

- Administering IV medication

General Advice

- When administering IV medication, it is important that you are familiar with the therapeutic use of the drug and the possible side effects
- Ensure that the patient has no known drug allergies, that you obtain verbal consent and that you wear gloves
- Check the prescription and if you have any concerns, check with the prescriber

Equipment Checklist

(remember to check expiry dates on all equipment)

a) Tray: either single-use, disposable sterilised tray, or a decontaminated plastic tray that is cleaned pre/post procedure

b) Non-sterile gloves

c) Skin cleansing solution

d) Prescribed IV drug

e) 10 mL 0.9% saline for flush

f) Giving set (if required)

g) 2 x 21-gauge needle (or filter needle)

h) 1 x 10 mL syringe

i) 1 x syringe (size depending on medication)

j) Sharps bin: the sharps bin should always be taken to the point of care

Administering IV Medication

Checks and Preparation

1. Introduce yourself to the patient and obtain consent
2. Check the patient's name, hospital number, date of birth
3. Check the prescriber's signature
4. Check the prescription dose, date, time and route of admission
5. Check the allergy status of the patient
6. Check the batch number and expiry date of the medication and flush
7. Check medication for discolouration or cloudiness
8. Check that the patient has a patent IV cannula in situ
9. Check that the cannula site has no sign of infection or phlebitis
10. Collect the equipment you require
11. Wash hands, don non-sterile gloves

Ensure you follow Trust policy for checking IV medication, usually it should be checked by two qualified healthcare professionals, to ensure patient safely

Giving an IV Injection

1. Clean the coloured port of the cannula using skin cleansing solution
2. Check the cannula is patent by flushing (assembled as previously described) 5 mL of 0.9% saline through the port (Fig 4.13)
3. Tap the medication ampoule to dislodge any medication at the neck and snap open
4. Draw up the correct volume of medication using a needle and syringe
    *   If the medication is in a glass vial, use a filter needle to draw up the medication to avoid aspiration of glass shards
    *   If the medication is in a powder, reconstitute the solution following the manufacturer's guidelines
5. Tap the syringe to dislodge any air bubbles to the top of the syringe. Immediately dispose of any sharps
6. Expel any air that is left in the syringe and dispose of the needle in the sharps bin
7. Attach the syringe to the cannula and administer the IV medication as directed by the drug manufactures guidelines
8. Flush the cannula with the remaining 5 mL of 0.9% saline
9. Check the cannula site

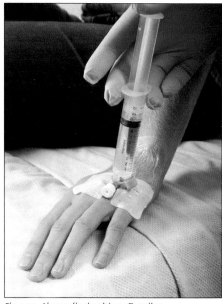

Fig 4.13: Always flush with 0.9% saline

Giving an IV Infusion

1. Complete an IV additive label (available from the pharmacy) and attach it to the fluid bag. (Fig 4.14) The label must state:
    *   The patient's name, hospital number and date of birth
    *   The name, dose and batch number of the medication
    *   The expiry date of the medication
    *   The date and time the medication was added to the bag
    *   The signatures of the healthcare professionals administering and checking the medication
2. Clean the injection port on the fluid bag with skin cleansing solution
3. Inject the medication into the fluid bag via the injection port
4. Dispose of sharps
5. Gently turn the fluid bag upside down several time to mix the drug with the fluid. Cleans cannula port
6. Follow the instructions as outlined in station 3.7 (to prepare the fluid and giving set). Once completed, hang the IV fluid bag up on a drip stand and allow the fluid to run through into the cannula
7. Hang the IV fluid bag and calculate the flow rate as directed by the prescription

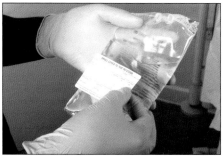

Fig 4.14: An example of an additive label

Finishing

1. Sign the drug chart stating the date and time that the medication was given
2. Monitor the patient's observations to ensure that there is no acute reaction

---

Mark Scheme for Examiner

Introduction and General Advice

Introduces self (clean hands) ☐ ☐ ☐ ☐ ☐

Identifies patient (3 points of ID) ☐ ☐ ☐ ☐ ☐

Explains procedure, identifies concerns and obtains consent ☐ ☐ ☐ ☐ ☐

Checks allergies ☐ ☐ ☐ ☐ ☐

Preparation

Obtains equipment and checks expiry dates ☐ ☐ ☐ ☐ ☐

Washes hands, dons non-sterile gloves ☐ ☐ ☐ ☐ ☐

Attaches syringe to needle for drawing up medication

Checks prescription

Checks medication and flush

Checks cannula site

IV Injection

Draws up flush and checks cannula patency

Checks cannula patency

Opens ampoule and draws up medication

Expels air

Gives medication through cannula

Flushes cannula

Checks cannula site

IV Infusion

Completes IV additive label

Cleans injection port

Injects medication into fluid bag. Disposes of sharps

Mixes medication and fluid

Cleans cannula port

Sets up the IV giving set

Calculates the drip rate

Finishing

Sign and date the patient's drug chart

Disposes of equipment and cleans tray

Removes gloves and washes hands

Assesses patient to ensure no acute drug reaction

General Points

Talks throughout the procedure to the patient

Avoids patient contamination (i.e. NTT)

Questions and Answers for Candidate

Additional Questions to Consider

What are the possible complications of IV administration of medication?

- Phlebitis
- Extravasion into soft tissue
- Air embolism
- Drug reaction

1. What are the benefits of giving a drug IV?
2. What is a Hickman line and when might it be used?
3. What would you do if you accidentally gave the wrong dose of an IV medication?

Station 6: DRUG ADMINISTRATION VIA NEBULISER

Mr Netherby is a 49-year-old man with known chronic asthma. He has presented to hospital with shortness of breath, inability to speak in full sentences, tachycardia and tachypnoea. You have been asked to give Mr Netherby salbutamol via a nebuliser.

Objectives

- Learning the indications for administering nebulised medication
- Administering medication via a nebuliser

General Advice

When administering any medication, it is important to ensure:
- The patient has no known drug allergies
- That you gain verbal consent
- That you wear gloves

Equipment Checklist

(remember to check expiry dates on all equipment)

a) Tray: either single-use, disposable sterilised tray, or a decontaminated plastic tray that is cleaned pre/post procedure
b) Non-sterile gloves
c) Oxygen mask (check the prescription chart for which mask should be used)
d) Oxygen tubing
e) 10 mL syringe (to draw up medication. Requires additional equipment for preparing medication depending on specific drug e.g. 0.9% saline)
f) Prescribed oxygen
g) Prescribed medication

Procedure

1. Wash hands and don a pair of non-sterile gloves
2. Position the patient upright, if possible
3. Check the expiry date of the medication
4. Draw up the prescribed medication into a sterile syringe Place the medication into the nebuliser. Note whether the patient is to have their medication through oxygen or just air. If oxygen is prescribed, connect the nebuliser to oxygen tubing
5. Ensure that mist is being released from the mask, indicating that the nebuliser is working
6. Apply the face mask to the patient. Instruct the patient to breathe normally through their mouth (Fig 4.15)
7. Dispose of the syringe
8. Document the drug administration in the drug chart
9. Assess the patient for adverse effects to the medication
10. Ensure mask and chamber are rinsed and air dried after each use

Indication for administering medication via a nebuliser:
- To administer medication when a patient is unable to effectively use inhalers
- To administer mucolytics to aid expectoration
- To administer antibiotics e.g. in some cases of cystic fibrosis

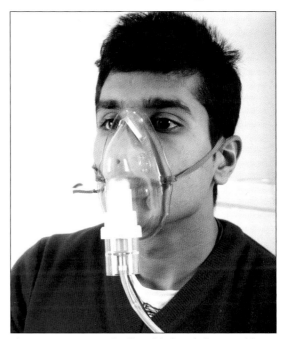

Fig 4.15: Ensure you are familiar with the nebulisers used in your trust

'In the majority of patients in an acute setting, it is best to use a non-rebreather mask if the type of oxygen mask has not been specified on the oxygen prescription chart. Do note, however, that in some patients, such as those with COPD, you may need to accurately control the amount of oxygen delivered with the nebuliser. This can be achieved using a Venturi mask'

Mark Scheme for Examiner

Introduction and General Advice
Introduces self (clean hands) ☐ ☐ ☐ ☐ ☐

Identifies patient (3 points of ID) ☐ ☐ ☐ ☐ ☐

Explains procedure, identifies concerns and obtains consent ☐ ☐ ☐ ☐ ☐

Checks for allergies ☐ ☐ ☐ ☐ ☐

Preparation
Obtains equipment, medication and checks expiry dates ☐ ☐ ☐ ☐ ☐

Washes hands, dons non-sterile gloves ☐ ☐ ☐ ☐ ☐

Positions the patient upright ☐ ☐ ☐ ☐ ☐

Administering Medication
Draws up medication ☐ ☐ ☐ ☐ ☐

Places medication in the nebuliser ☐ ☐ ☐ ☐ ☐

Connects facemask, nebuliser and oxygen ☐ ☐ ☐ ☐ ☐

Applies face mask, and asks the patient to breath normally ☐ ☐ ☐ ☐ ☐

Finishing
Monitors the patient ☐ ☐ ☐ ☐ ☐

Signs the patient's drug chart ☐ ☐ ☐ ☐ ☐

Disposes of equipment and cleans tray ☐ ☐ ☐ ☐ ☐

Removes gloves and washes hands ☐ ☐ ☐ ☐ ☐

General Points
Talks throughout the procedure to the patient ☐ ☐ ☐ ☐ ☐

Ensures patient comfort ☐ ☐ ☐ ☐ ☐

Questions and Answers for Candidate

What medication might be administered via a nebuliser?

- ß-agonists
- Mucolytics
- Anticholinergics
- Antibiotics
- Antimicrobials (e.g. pentamidine for pneumocystis pneumonia)
- Adrenaline

Additional Questions to Consider

1. What are the indications for giving salbutamol via a nebuliser instead of inhalers?
2. How should nebulisers be maintained and cleaned?
3. What features would support a diagnosis of severe asthma?
4. What triggers could potentially cause an asthma exacerbation?
5. Can patients have nebulisers at home?

Station 7: OPERATING A SYRINGE DRIVER

Mrs Peach is a 79-year-old woman who has known metastatic breast cancer. She has been admitted to hospital with pneumonia and uncontrolled pain. She has been deteriorating and is now unable to swallow tablets. The patient, along with her family and the medical team, have made a decision that she will receive supportive care only. Please discuss the use of syringe drivers with the examiner.

Objectives

- To know the indications for commencing a syringe driver
- To understand the general principles of operating a syringe driver

Explaining a Syringe Driver to the Patient

1. A syringe driver is a small portable pump that supplies medication continuously via a line attached to a syringe
2. Syringe drivers are useful when patients find tablets hard to swallow. Instead, a small needle or plastic tube is placed just underneath your skin; which allows the medication to enter the body
3. Several different drugs can be put through the syringe driver to help with symptoms such as pain, nausea and vomiting
4. Medication is supplied throughout the 24 hour period, helping to consistently control symptoms, as the amount of each drug in the bloodstream should remain constant
5. Although the skin at the site of the needle can get wet, the pump itself should be kept dry

General Principles to Consider when Operating a Syringe Driver

There are currently many different types of syringe drivers used in hospitals. Ensure that you familiarise yourself and have training with the particular model used in your Trust. Some automatically calculate the infusion rates whilst others require the infusion rate to be set manually (Fig 4.16)

- When drawing up medication for a syringe driver, the drugs should be checked by two members of the nursing/medical staff using the prescription chart
- Some Trusts permit single nurse administration as long as no controlled drugs are used
- Each syringe used should be labelled with the patient's name, date of birth, the names and doses of drugs, diluent, total volume, time, date and signatures of those preparing the medication
- Each syringe should carry enough medication for 24 hours
- Syringe drivers are locked inside a plastic cage to ensure that they cannot be tampered with. The nurse in charge usually holds the key to the cage
- Most syringe drivers are battery powered and the batteries can often be changed whilst the driver is locked inside the plastic cage

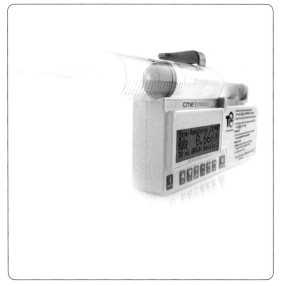

Fig 4.16: T34™ Ambulatory Syringe Pump. Common component parts are found on all syringe drivers but ensure you are familiar with those used in your Trust

Inserting the Metal Needle or Plastic Cannula

There are different types of giving sets in use. Metal needles are more commonly found in hospitals and the community, whereas plastic cannulae are more commonly found in hospices. Please ensure you are familiar with the type of giving set used in your Trust

Equipment Checklist

(remember to check expiry dates on all equipment)

a) Tray: either single-use, disposable sterilised tray, or a decontaminated plastic tray that is cleaned pre/post procedure
b) 2 x non-sterile gloves
c) Skin cleansing solution
d) Metal needle or cannula
e) Infusion line and giving set
f) Syringe driver
g) Battery
h) Medication in labelled syringe
i) Clear film dressing
j) Lockable box (if used)
k) Carry case (if used)

Setting Up the Syringe Driver

1. Obtain consent
2. Wash hands and put on non-sterile gloves
3. Make up the medication solution as prescribed in an appropriately sized syringe
4. Prime the line and giving set in accordance with manufacturers' instructions and attach the syringe to the syringe driver
5. Confirm patient identity in accordance with Trust policy
6. Locate an insertion site. The giving set can be inserted subcutaneously in a site with adipose tissue, providing it is not inflamed, or oedematous. Avoid using areas where radiotherapy is targeted. The site of insertion should be checked at least once a day for inflammation, soreness, hardening of the skin or infection. If any of these are seen, the site should be changed immediately. Sites used commonly are:
   - Upper arm
   - Abdomen
   - Chest
   - Thigh
7. Wash your hands and put on new pair of non-sterile gloves
8. Clean the area of insertion using skin cleansing solution
9. Insert the needle or cannula into the skin at an angle of 45° and cover with clear film dressing to secure in place
10. Set the pump to run at the correct rate
11. Put in lockable box or carry case (if used)
12. Remove gloves and wash hands
13. Document the date, time, rate of infusion, battery status and insertion site in the patient's notes
14. Sign the patient's drug chart

Drugs Commonly Used in Syringe Drivers for Palliation

Not all drugs are compatible with each other, so it is important to check with the Palliative Care Team or the Palliative Care Formulary whether the drug combination you wish to use is permissible.

Although water is usually recommended to dilute medication, normal saline must be used with diclofenac, ketorolac and ketamine.

Drug	Indication	Important Information
Cyclizine	Nausea Vomiting	Can cause insertion site inflammation; this can be helped by diluting the drug well with 'Water for Injections'
Dexamethasone	Antiemetic Pain Raised intracranial pressure	Advisable to put in a separate syringe driver in larger doses instead of mixing it with another drug
Diamorphine	Pain Shortness of breath Cough	Mixes well with most drugs
Haloperidol	Nausea Vomiting Hiccups	Extrapyramidal side effects can occur with high doses
Hyoscine hydrobromide	Excess secretion	Mixes well with most drugs
Metoclopramide	Nausea Vomiting Delayed gastric emptying	Mixes well with most drugs
Midazolam	Agitation Epilepsy Muscle spasm	Mixes well with most drugs

'If you have any worries or concerns regarding syringe drivers, the hospital palliative care team members are usually available for advice. If the prescription for the syringe driver changes, the original syringe should be discarded and a new syringe and infusion line of medication prepared'

Mark Scheme for Examiner

Introduction and General Advice

Introduces self (clean hands) ☐ ☐ ☐ ☐ ☐

Identifies patient (3 points of ID) ☐ ☐ ☐ ☐ ☐

Explains procedure, identifies concerns and obtains consent ☐ ☐ ☐ ☐ ☐

Checks for allergies ☐ ☐ ☐ ☐ ☐

Setting Up the Syringe Driver

Washes hands and dons non-sterile gloves ☐ ☐ ☐ ☐ ☐

Obtains equipment, medication and checks expiry dates ☐ ☐ ☐ ☐ ☐

Makes up medication in appropriate sized syringe. Labels each syringe correctly ☐ ☐ ☐ ☐ ☐

Primes the line and giving set with the medication ☐ ☐ ☐ ☐ ☐

Attaches syringe to syringe driver ☐ ☐ ☐ ☐ ☐

Inserting the Metal Needle or Plastic Cannula

Locates appropriate site for insertion ☐ ☐ ☐ ☐ ☐

Washes hands, dons non-sterile gloves, and cleans insertion site ☐ ☐ ☐ ☐ ☐

Inserts the needle or cannula ☐ ☐ ☐ ☐ ☐

Sets rate on syringe driver ☐ ☐ ☐ ☐ ☐

Covers needle/cannula with clear dressing ☐ ☐ ☐ ☐ ☐

Finishing

Tells the patient to inform a member of staff if they feel unwell or have any problems with the insertion site ☐ ☐ ☐ ☐ ☐

Signs the patient's drug chart ☐ ☐ ☐ ☐ ☐

Disposes of equipment and cleans tray ☐ ☐ ☐ ☐ ☐

Removes gloves and washes hands ☐ ☐ ☐ ☐ ☐

General Points

Talks throughout the procedure to the patient ☐ ☐ ☐ ☐ ☐

Ensures patient comfort ☐ ☐ ☐ ☐ ☐

MEDICATION ADMINISTRATION

Questions and Answers for Candidate

What are some indications for syringe driver use?

- Patients with nausea or vomiting
- Patients with dysphagia
- Patients who are too weak to swallow tablets
- Patients with oral tumours or infections
- Unconscious patients
- Poor patient compliance with other mechanisms of drug administration
- Poor alimentary absorption
- Patients with no intravenous access

What are you looking for when assessing the insertion site of a syringe driver?

- Metal needle or plastic cannula in situ
- Erythema
- Swelling
- Warmth
- Pain or tenderness

Additional Questions to Consider

1. What are the advantages of using a syringe driver rather than injections?

2. Why might you give hyoscine hydrobromide? What patients might particularly benefit from it?

3. A patient with advanced pancreatic cancer is felt to be dying, and is on palliative treatment. They are on a low dose of morphine through the syringe driver, but are still in pain. Discuss how you would manage their pain

5 MEDICINE AND SURGERY

MEDICINE AND SURGERY

Station 1: SIMPLE DRESSING CHANGE

Mrs Clifton is a 62-year-old woman who is under your care following a laparotomy. It has been two days since her operation. Please change her abdominal dressing.

Objectives

- Undertake a simple dressing change

General Advice

- Simple dressing changes are sterile procedures
- The type of dressing required depends on the nature and size of the wound
- Most wounds are documented in the nursing notes. Ensure you are familiar with your Trust's policy on documenting wounds and wound management
- Clinical photography is useful to document wounds

Equipment Checklist

(remember to check expiry dates on all equipment) (Fig 5.1)

a) Tray: either single-use, disposable sterilised tray, or a decontaminated plastic tray that is cleaned pre/post procedure

b) 2 x sterile gloves

c) Single use apron

d) Gauze

e) Sterile water or saline

f) Universal sterile container

g) Sterile scissors

h) Tape

i) Surgical dressing

j) Clinical waste bag

k) Optional: prescribed topical agent, steri-strips

Simple Dressing Change

Preparation

1. Introduce yourself to the patient and obtain verbal consent
2. Adequately expose the wound area
3. Place the clinical waste bag within reach
4. Apply single use apron
5. Wash hands and don gloves
6. Prepare items required for dressing change:
   - Open any packaging
   - Cut dressings to size using sterile scissors (Fig 5.2)
   - Cut tape to size
   - Pour sterile water or normal saline into universal container
   - Place initials and date on the dressing or tape
7. Remove the old dressing and place it in the clinical waste bag

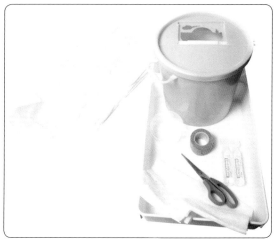

Fig 5.1: This is a sterile procedure so ensure you have all the equipment you require before going to the patient

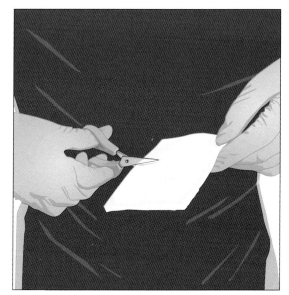

Fig 5.2: Cut using sterile scissors

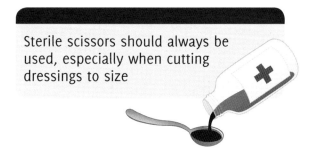

Sterile scissors should always be used, especially when cutting dressings to size

Assessing the Wound

1. Assess the wound for:
   - Size
   - Colour
   - Surrounding erythema
   - Temperature
   - Odour
   - Discharge
2. Compare your findings with those documented in the notes
3. Document your findings in the patient notes

'If there are any new changes to the wound such as discharge or odour, this may indicate an infection. It is important to swab such wounds and alert the patient's medical team'

Changing the Dressing

1. Wash hands and don sterile gloves
2. Clean the wound with sterile water or normal saline using a washout technique
3. Pat the skin surrounding the wound dry with gauze
4. If any cream or ointment has been prescribed, apply using clean gauze as per drug chart
5. Cover the wound with a new surgical dressing
6. Remove gloves and place all soiled items into the clinical waste bag
7. Document the dressing change in the patient's notes

'If the dressing seems stuck when attempting to remove it from the patient, try moistening the edges with sterile water or normal saline to ease removal'

Summary of Dressings

Dressing	Indication for Use
Film dressing	• Primary dressing
	• Secondary dressing
	• Protection from friction/shearing force
Absorbent dressing	• Wound with exudates
Moist dressing	• Dry wound with slough
	• Necrotic wound
Non-adherent dressing	• Wound with new granulation tissue
Simple island dressing	• Wound with sutures

MEDICINE AND SURGERY

Mark Scheme for Examiner

Introduction and General Advice

Introduces self (clean hands)

Identifies patient (3 points of ID)

Explains procedure, identifies concerns and obtains consent

Checks allergies if giving medication

Preparation

Obtains equipment and checks expiry dates

Applies single use apron

Washes hands, dons sterile gloves

Prepares equipment

Exposes wound by removing old dressing

Ensures the dressing is the correct size

Assessing the Wound

Comments on: size, colour, erythema, temperature, odour, discharge

Compares findings with those previously documented

Documents findings

Dressing Change

Washes hands and dons new pair of gloves

Cleans the wound

Dries surrounding skin and applies any medications

Applies new dressing

Finishing

Tells patient to inform staff if wound becomes painful

Documents dressing change in patient notes

Disposes of equipment and cleans tray

Removes gloves and washes hands

General Points

Talks throughout the procedure to patient

Avoids patient contamination (i.e. NTT)

Questions and Answers for Candidate

Give three signs of a wound infection

- Slow healing
- Erythema
- Increasing pain
- Discharge
- Swelling
- Pyrexia

What factors can negatively affect wound healing?

- Age
- Stress
- Diabetes
- Medication e.g. steroids
- Obesity
- Smoking
- Poor nutrition
- Infection
- Inflammation
- Ischaemia

What is the difference between a primary and secondary dressing?

- A primary dressing is one that is placed directly on a wound. A secondary dressing is one that is used to hold a primary dressing in place

Additional Questions to Consider

1. When is a tetanus injection indicated?
2. What is the difference between primary intention and secondary intention healing?
3. When might you involve specialists in managing a wound?
4. What is the role of a tissue viability nurse?
5. What medical conditions can cause delayed healing?

Station 2: SPIROMETRY

Mrs Melini is a 55-year-old woman with a 30 pack year smoking history. She has come to your clinic complaining of a recurrent productive cough and breathlessness. Perform spirometry and interpret the results.

Objectives

- Learn how to perform spirometry
- Measure the Forced Expiratory Volume in 1 second (FEV1), Forced Vital Capacity (FVC) and interpret their results

General Advice

- Ensure that you have introduced yourself, identified the patient and washed your hands

Explaining the Procedure to the Patient

- The spirometer is a machine that measures how well your lungs are working
- It gives information such as whether your lungs are expanding sufficiently or whether your airways are narrowed thereby causing an obstruction to the flow of air out of the lungs
- I will demonstrate how to use the spirometer first and then you can have a couple of practice attempts before the readings are actually taken
- If you feel faint or light headed, just stop and breathe normally

> 'There are many different spirometers on the market; ensure you are familiar with the one you are about to use. Some patients may feel light headed whilst performing spirometry. It is therefore recommended that the patient is seated during the procedure'

Equipment Checklist (Fig 5.3)

a) Spirometer
b) Disposable mouth piece

How to Perform Spirometry

1. Ask the patient to relax and sit up straight
2. Attach a clean mouthpiece to the spirometer
3. Ask the patient to breathe in as deeply as they can
4. Instruct the patient to breathe out as hard and as fast as possible, until their lungs are empty
5. Repeat the procedure a further two more times
6. Ask the patient to perform the procedure without instruction to check understanding and technique

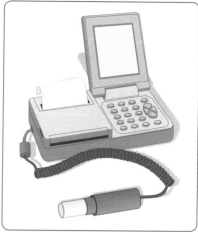

Fig 5.3: Spirometer and mouth piece

'Ensure the age, sex and height of the patient has been recorded in order to calculate the predicted FEV₁ and FVC. The best two readings should be within 100mL or 5% of each other'

Obstructive disorder, such as asthma and COPD: (Fig 5.4)
- FEV1 is reduced to < 80% of the predicted value
- FVC is often reduced but to a lesser extent than FEV1
- FEV1/FVC ratio is reduced to <0.7

Restrictive disorder, such as idiopathic pulmonary fibrosis and asbestosis: (Fig 5.5)
- FEV1 is reduced to < 80% of the predicted value
- FVC is reduced to < 80% of the predicted value
- FEV1/FVC ratio is > 0.7

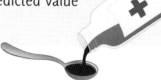

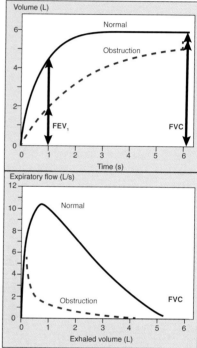

Fig 5.4: Typical spirometry findings in obstruction

You can distinguish further between different causes of lung disease with abnormal spirometry using a formal set of pulmonary function tests. It is most commonly used to help investigate restrictive pattern spirometry. One of the most important pieces of information gathered from these tests is the measurement of the diffusion capacity of the lung; this looks at how readily oxygen can diffuse from the alveoli to the blood by measuring the difference between inspired and expired carbon monoxide. It is represented as 'DLCO' (Diffusion capacity of the lung for carbon monoxide) or 'TLCO' (Transfer factor of the lung for carbon monoxide). It is decreased in any condition that affects the effective alveolar surface area

Causes of a decreased DLCO:
- Interstitial lung disease
- Pneumonitis
- Sarcoidosis
- Asbestosis
- Miliary TB
- Heart failure

Causes of an increased DLCO:
- Polycythaemia
- Pulmonary haemorrhage
- Left to right intracardiac shunt
- Morbid obesity

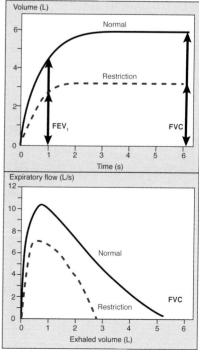

Fig 5.5: Typical spirometry findings in restriction

Present your Findings

Mrs Melini is a 55-year-old woman complaining of a recurrent cough and shortness of breath. Spirometry reveals that she has an FEV1 of 75% of her predicted value and an FEV1 to FVC ratio of 0.65. This is in keeping with a mild obstructive disorder. Given the nature of her symptoms and her heavy smoking history, this is most like to be COPD

Mark Scheme for Examiner

Introduction and General Advice

Introduces self (clean hands)

Identifies patient (3 points of ID)

Ensures that consent has been taken

Explains procedure, identifies concerns

Explaining Spirometry

Describes the technique of using the spirometer (breathe deeply, then breathe out as hard and fast as possible into the mouthpiece until lungs are empty)

Mentions it should be done three times

Watches the patient do it without instruction

Records the patient's age, sex and height

Finishing the Consultation

Elicits patient concerns and questions

Arranges a follow up appointment if necessary or offers contact details

Thanks the patient and close the consultation

General Points

Checks patient understanding throughout the consultation, avoiding medical jargon, and offers information leaflets

Maintains good eye contact, is polite and engaging with the patient

MEDICINE AND SURGERY

Questions and Answers for Candidate

Additional Questions to Consider

Give some reasons for inconsistent readings during spirometry

- Inadequate or incomplete inhalation
- Lips not tight around the mouthpiece
- Exhalation stops before complete expiration
- Coughing

How is the severity of airflow obstruction graded?

- Mild obstruction - FEV1 between 50–80%
- Moderate obstruction - FEV1 between 30–49%
- Severe obstruction - FEV1 <30% predicted

1. What are the management strategies of COPD?

2. How is an acute exacerbation of COPD treated in the hospital setting?

3. List five causes of restrictive lung disease

Station 3: KNEE JOINT ASPIRATION

Mr Jenner is a 62-year-old man who presented to hospital with an acutely swollen left knee. On examination, he is pyrexial and his knee is tender, swollen and erythematous with reduced movement. This is the first time the patient has had any trouble with any of his joints. Please perform a diagnostic aspiration of his knee joint.

Objectives

- Performing a knee joint aspiration

General Advice

- Ensure that your patient has given verbal consent for the procedure
- It is vital to check whether the patient has any known drug allergies to anaesthetic agents or bleeding disorders as it may be necessary to modify their medication prior to the procedure

Equipment Checklist

(remember to check expiry dates on all equipment) (Fig 5.6)

a) Tray: either single-use, disposable sterilised tray, or a decontaminated plastic tray that is cleaned pre/post procedure
b) Antiseptic solution
c) Sterile universal container
d) Sterile gloves
e) Single use apron
f) 10 mL syringe
g) 25-gauge needle and 2 x 21-gauge needles
h) 5-10 mL lidocaine 1%
i) 30-60 mL syringe
j) Towel
k) Specimen bottles
l) Gauze
m) Tape
n) Sharps bin: the sharps bin should always be taken to the point of care

Note: Skin cleansing solutions and method will vary depending on local policy

Performing a Knee Joint Aspiration (lateral approach)

Preparation

1. Ask the patient to lie on the bed and expose their knee
2. Place a rolled-up towel under their knee joint so it is slightly flexed
3. Palpate the margins of the knee joint including the patella and medial joint line
4. Locate the intended puncture site, which is the intersection point between the lateral and proximal borders of the patella (Fig 5.7)
5. Pour antiseptic solution into the universal container
6. Wash hands, don apron and sterile gloves
7. Clean site using gauze soaked in antiseptic solution, from the intended site of puncture outwards. Allow to fully dry
8. Attach the 21-gauge needle to the 10mL syringe and draw-up 5-10mL of lidocaine 1%. Change to the 25-gauge needle
9. Infiltrate 2-4ml of lidocaine 1% into the knee joint at the intended puncture site. This is done by slowly inserting the needle whilst concurrently aspirating back to ensure you have not hit a blood vessel

What are the indications for performing a knee joint aspiration?
Diagnostic:
- Septic arthritis
- Gout
- Pseudogout
Therapeutic:
- Effusion
- Haemarthrosis

Additionally, medication (such as steroids) can be injected into the joint to assist in the treatment of tendonitis or bursitis

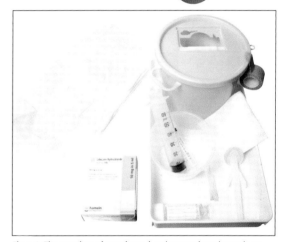

Fig 5.6: The number of specimen bottles requires depends on the investigations you are going to order. It is better to fill too many bottles that not have enough

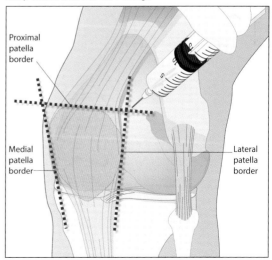

Proximal patella border

Medial patella border

Lateral patella border

Fig 5.7: Note the important anatomical landmarks (labelled) when aspirating a knee joint

Aspiration

1. Attach the second 21-gauge needle to the 30-60mL syringe
2. Insert the needle into the soft tissue between the patella and femur at the intended puncture site
3. Direct the needle at a 45° angle towards the midline of the medial side of the joint
4. Once correctly in place, aspirate the synovial fluid
5. Once the syringe is full with synovial fluid, remove the needle and syringe from the knee joint
6. Apply pressure to the puncture site using gauze and secure with tape
7. Dispose of needle in the sharps bin
8. Transfer the fluid into the specimen bottles and label at the bedside
9. Inform the patient to let a member of staff know if the site is painful, bleeds, or if they have any other concerns
10. Explain that they can remove the dressing after a couple of hours
11. Remove gloves and wash hands
12. Document the procedure in the patient's notes

> There are several different techniques for performing knee joint aspiration. The commonest is the lateral approach described above. Others include the medial approach, which involves entering the joint under the middle of the patella, or the anterior approach

Mark Scheme for Examiner

Introduction and General Advice

Introduces self (clean hands)

Identifies patient (3 points of ID)

Explains procedure, identifies concerns and obtains consent

Checks for allergies, needle phobia and clotting

Preparation

Obtains equipment and checks expiry dates

Prepares equipment

Positions the patient

Locates site of needle insertion

Washes hands, dons sterile gloves and apron

Cleans site

Prepares LA

Infiltrates intended puncture site with LA

Aspiration

Inserts needle and syringe

Aspirates synovial fluid

Disposes of sharp immediately

Applies dressing over puncture site

Finishing

Tells patient to inform staff if site becomes painful or bleeds and that they can remove dressing after a few hours

Transfers fluid into specimen bottles, labels at bedside

Disposes of equipment and clean tray

Removes gloves and wash hands

Documents procedure in the patient notes

General Points

Talks throughout the procedure to the patient

Avoids patient contamination (i.e. NTT)

Questions and Answers for Candidate

Give two causes of haemarthrosis

- Trauma
- Haemophilia and other coagulation disorders
- Anticoagulant therapy

Additional Questions to Consider

1. What is the management of septic arthritis?
2. What are the risk factors for gout?
3. How would you diagnose a crystal arthopathy?
4. How would you treat a haemarthrosis?

Station 4: NASOGASTRIC TUBE INSERTION

Mrs Tregony is an 84-year-old woman who has been admitted following a stroke. She has been fully assessed and your consultant has asked you to insert a NG tube as she has an impaired swallow. Please perform a NG tube insertion and describe how you would assess the position of the tube.

Objectives

- Performing NG tube insertion
- Checking NG tube positioning

General Advice

- Ensure that your patient has consented to the procedure and there are no contraindications to NG tube insertion

Equipment Checklist

(remember to check expiry dates on all equipment) (Fig 5.8)

a) Non-sterile gloves
b) Disposable plastic apron
c) Lubricant gel
d) NG tube
e) 60 mL syringe
f) pH strip
g) Sticky tape
h) Drainage system
i) Cup of water
Optional - LA spray

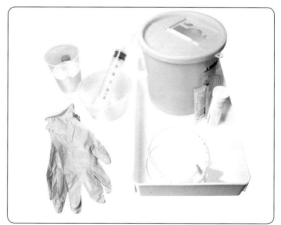

Fig 5.8: Collect all your equipment prior to starting the procedure. It may be helpful to have an assistant

Before starting the procedure ensure you select the correct size for the patient. NG tubes come in various sizes: 8 - 18 Fr. Tube size selection depends on the patient's build and reason for insertion

Inserting a NG Tube

Preparation

1. Introduce yourself to the patient and check consent
2. Ensure the patient has no allergies to anaesthetic spray (if this is being used)
3. Sit the patient upright with their chin up
4. Estimate the length of tube required by measuring from the tip of the patient's nose to the xiphisternum passing via the tragus of the ear (Fig 5.9)
5. Wash hands and don gloves and apron

NG Tube Insertion

1. Lubricate the end 5-8cms of the tube with lubricant gel
2. Slide the tube along the floor of the nasal cavity initially aiming towards the occiput. There is usually slight resistance as the tube passes into the oesophagus (Fig 5.10)
3. Ask the patient to repeatedly swallow or offer sips of water to assist with tube insertion
4. Advance the tube to the pre-determined distance, and then aspirate stomach fluid using the syringe
5. Assess the positioning of the tube using pH indicator paper
6. Tape the tube securely to the patient's nose and document length of tube inserted at nostril entry point
7. Attach tube to a drainage system or spigot off as directed

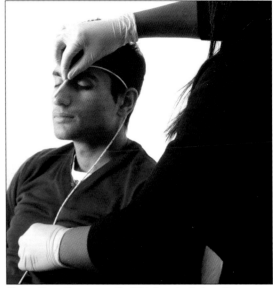

Fig 5.9: Correctly measure the NG tube prior to insertion

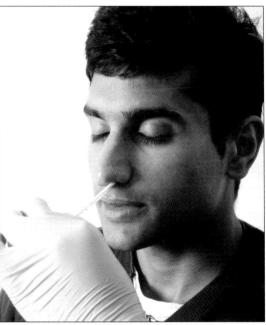

Fig 5.10: Constantly talk to the patient when inserting an NG tube

Anaesthetic throat spray can be used prior to the insertion of the NG tube, however it can result in an unsafe swallow; therefore, asking patients to subsequently swallow sips of water can be dangerous. Patients should not have anything to eat or drink for at least one hour following the use of anaesthetic throat spray

Verifying the Correct Position

Method 1 – pH Testing
(usually a safe method if the tube is only being used for drainage)

1. Aspirate the contents of the NG tube using a sterile oral syringe
2. Place a small amount of the aspirated contents on pH indicator paper
3. Check the pH reading (Fig 5.11)

If the patient coughs excessively, the tube could be incorrectly placed. Withdraw the tube and attempt to repeat the insertion

There are several substances that can affect the pH of the stomach contents: recent intake of milk, proton pump inhibitors and H2 receptor antagonists. These should be taken into account when interpreting the pH result

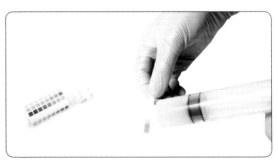

Fig 5.11: pH testing must be undertaken before an NG tube can be used

MEDICINE AND SURGERY

Method 2 – Chest X-ray: must always be used when the tube is for feeding
(refer to local guidelines for current policies)

- This method is indicated if the pH reading is › 5.5 or if there is any doubt with regards to the position of the NG tube

- A chest X-ray including the upper abdomen is required to locate the tip of the NG tube (which is radio-opaque)

Finishing

1. Remove the guidewire (if NG tube has one)
2. Fix the tube in place using tape
3. Remove gloves and wash hands
4. Inform the patient that the procedure is complete and to speak to a member of staff if they feel any discomfort or have any further questions
5. Document the procedure in the patient's notes

Mark Scheme for Examiner

Introduction and General Advice

Introduces self (clean hands)   ☐ ☐ ☐ ☐ ☐

Identifies patient (3 points of ID)   ☐ ☐ ☐ ☐ ☐

Explains procedure, identifies concerns, checks allergies, and obtains consent   ☐ ☐ ☐ ☐ ☐

Preparation

Obtains equipment and checks expiry dates   ☐ ☐ ☐ ☐ ☐

Positions the patient   ☐ ☐ ☐ ☐ ☐

Applies single use apron   ☐ ☐ ☐ ☐ ☐

Washes hands, dons non-sterile gloves   ☐ ☐ ☐ ☐ ☐

Estimates NG tube length   ☐ ☐ ☐ ☐ ☐

NG Tube Insertion

Lubricates tube   ☐ ☐ ☐ ☐ ☐

Slides tube along nasal cavity to pre-determined distance (asking patient to swallow during advancement)   ☐ ☐ ☐ ☐ ☐

Verifying Position – pH Testing

Aspirates contents   ☐ ☐ ☐ ☐ ☐

Assesses with pH paper   ☐ ☐ ☐ ☐ ☐

Verifying Position – Chest X-ray

Orders chest X-ray to identify position   ☐ ☐ ☐ ☐ ☐

Finishing

Removes the guidewire   ☐ ☐ ☐ ☐ ☐

Decompresses the stomach   ☐ ☐ ☐ ☐ ☐

Disposes of equipment   ☐ ☐ ☐ ☐ ☐

Removes gloves and washes hands   ☐ ☐ ☐ ☐ ☐

Documents procedure in the patient notes   ☐ ☐ ☐ ☐ ☐

General Points

Talks throughout the procedure to the patient   ☐ ☐ ☐ ☐ ☐

Questions and Answers for Candidate

What are the common indications for NG tube insertion?

- Feeding (supplement oral intake or where oral intake is not possible)
- To empty the upper gastro-intestinal tract (e.g. bowel obstruction)

What are the contraindications to NG tube insertion?

- Nasal trauma
- Base of skull fracture
- Post-operative upper gastro-intestinal surgery patient. If a patient requires an NG tube in this setting, it will be inserted at the time of surgery. If this needed to be replaced, for any reason, this should be discussed with the senior surgeons overseeing their care

When should the position of the NG tube be confirmed?

- Immediately after initial placement
- Following significant vomiting or coughing
- If the patient complains of significant pain

Additional Questions to Consider

1. What are the possible consequences of a misplaced NG tube?
2. How long can a tube stay in situ before needing to be replaced?
3. What other types of feeding tubes do you know about?
4. How might you be able to tell if the NG tube is in the wrong place?

Station 5: DIAGNOSTIC PLEURAL TAP

Mrs Haines is a 52-year-old woman who presents with shortness of breath, fatigue and bloating. She admits that she has had some weight loss and menstrual irregularities. The respiratory examination demonstrates stony dull percussion on the right side and shifting dullness on abdominal percussion. Subsequent radiological investigations demonstrate a right-sided pleural effusion. Pelvic examination reveals the presence of a mass. Please perform a diagnostic aspiration of the pleural effusion and then interpret the findings.

Objectives

- Perform a pleural tap
- Interpret the results

General Advice

- Obtain valid consent
- An USS should be performed as part of the assessment for a suspected pleural effusion
- British Thoracic Society guidelines currently recommend the use of bedside ultrasound guidance for any pleural procedures such as diagnostic pleural taps as it increases the likelihood of success and reduces the risk of adverse events

Explaining a Pleural Tap to the Patient

1. A pleural tap is a procedure that allows us to obtain a sample of fluid which has built up in the space between your lungs and ribs. It is usually performed under ultrasound guidance
2. LA is injected around the area of skin where the needle is inserted to numb the skin and provide some pain relief
3. The sample is then obtained by inserting a needle through the skin, and into the space between your ribs and lung

Continues overleaf...

Equipment Checklist

(remember to check expiry dates on all equipment)

a) Sterile gloves and single use apron
b) 3 x skin cleansing swabs
c) 25-gauge needle
d) 3 x 21-gauge needles
e) 10 mL syringe (for LA)
f) 50 mL syringe (for pleural aspirate)
g) Sterile pack with sterile towels and drape
h) 10 mL lidocaine 1%
i) Sterile dressing
j) Sticky tape
k) Sterile specimen bottles (usually three plus a glucose bottle)
l) Sharps bin

MEDICINE AND SURGERY

4. We will extract a sample of fluid and send it to the laboratory for testing

5. The needle is then removed and a dressing put over the area

6. We may need to obtain a chest X-ray afterwards (to check for any leakage of air from the lungs)

7. It is possible that a sample of fluid cannot be obtained using this method and this may mean that we need to perform the procedure using ultrasound guidance

Performing a Pleural Tap

Preparation

1. Introduce yourself to the patient and obtain valid consent

2. Assemble the equipment

3. Expose the patient from head to waist

4. Position the patient sitting upright on the bed with pillows on a nearby table to support their arms (Fig 5.12)

5. Listen to the chest to determine the site and size of the pleural effusion

6. Percuss the upper border of the effusion and choose a site one or two interspaces below that upper border, in the mid-clavicular line

7. Open the sterile pack and arrange all equipment into the sterile field using an aseptic technique

Aseptic Technique

1. Wash hands and don sterile gloves and apron

2. Attach the 21-gauge needle to the 10 mL syringe and draw up 5-10 mL of lidocaine 1%. Attach the 25-gauge needle, and keep one 21-gauge needle ready for deeper infiltration

3. Attach the third 21-gauge needle to a 50mL syringe ready for pleural aspiration

4. Place all needle/syringe sets in the sterile field

5. Put the drape on the patient with the open window over the target area

6. Mark the site and clean the area with skin cleansing swabs in a spiral pattern three times

7. Inject LA; use the 25-gauge needle to superficially anaesthetize the skin

8. Swap the 25-gauge with the 21-gauge needle and anaesthetize down to the pleura. Once anaesthetized, note needle depth, and then withdraw the needle and syringe, disposing into sharps bin. Then insert the 21-gauge needle (attached to the 50 mL syringe), **aspirating whilst advancing** the needle

9. Draw up 10-20 mL of pleural fluid (Fig 5.13)

10. Withdraw the needle and place into the sterile field

11. Apply pressure with a sterile dressing and then tape the dressing into place

12. Transfer the aspirate into a sterile universal container and send to the laboratory for:
    • Chemistry: protein, glucose, pH, LDH, amylase
    • Bacteriology: microscopy, culture and sensitivity (MC&S)

13. If indicated, consider sending the sample for:
    • Acid-fast staining (if tuberculosis is suspected)
    • Immunology (rheumatoid factor, anti-nuclear antibodies, complement)
    • Cytology

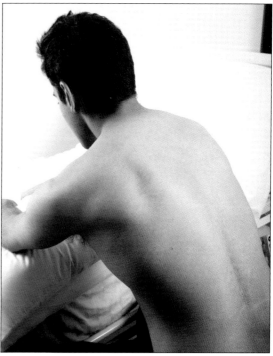

Fig 5.12: Correctly position the patient

'Pleural taps are usually performed under ultrasound guidance. It is advisable to stay at or above the 8th Intercostal space (T8) to avoid the liver or the spleen and to stay below the tip of the scapula by at least 2 inches'

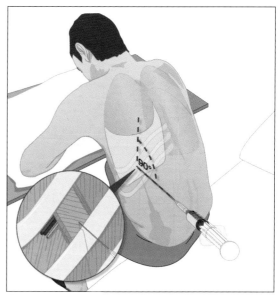

Fig 5.13: Correct positioning for pleural aspiration. The needle should be inserted perpendicular to the skin (drape not shown)

Venous Blood Sample

A venous blood sample can be taken for serum protein and LDH. This is to compare the protein and LDH in the pleural space with that in the blood (using Light's criteria), and determine whether the pleural aspirate is exudative or transudative. A capillary glucose is also helpful for this reason

Documenting the Procedure

Document under the following headings:
- Pleural tap performed
- Indications for the procedure
- Patient consent
- Relevant laboratory investigations (e.g. INR/ prothrombin time (PT), platelet count)
- Procedure technique, sterile preparation, anaesthetic and amount used, amount of fluid obtained, appearance of fluid obtained, estimated blood loss
- Complications
- Subsequent tests ordered, if any, e.g. chest X-ray/CT/ultrasound scan (USS)

- All needles should be inserted perpendicular to the skin directly above the upper edge of the corresponding rib into the pleural space occupied by the pleural fluid
  - o This minimizes the risk of the needle damaging the neurovascular bundle, which runs along the underside of the rib
- Whilst advancing the needle during deep LA infiltration, make sure to aspirate regularly. Stop when you aspirate fluid, as this indicates that you have reached the pleural space
- If the patient feels faint during the procedure, stop and withdraw the needle immediately and lie the patient down
  - o This may be avoided by administering adequate local anaesthesia

Risks of Performing a Pleural Tap

Common (>5%)	Uncommon (1 – 5%)	Rare (Less than 1%)
• Pneumothorax	• Pain	• Haemothorax
• Infection (wound or chest)	• Shortness of breath	• Damage to nearby structures (i.e. liver, spleen, colon)
• Coughing		• Death
• Fainting (vasovagal)		

MEDICINE AND SURGERY

Interpreting a Pleural Aspirate (without comparison to blood sample values)

Transudate (protein <30g/L)	Exudative (protein >30g/L)
Caused by the 'failures' and low protein states • Liver failure/cirrhosis • Heart failure • Nephrotic syndrome • Hypothyroidism • Fluid overload • Meig's syndrome	• Pneumonia • Tuberculosis (TB) • Malignancy • Pulmonary embolism

Guideline:

Pleural Disease Guideline, British Thoracic Society, 2010 http://www.brit-thoracic.org.uk/Portals/0/ Guidelines/PleuralDiseaseGuidelines/Pleural%20Guideline%202010/PleuralDiseaseQRG_web.pdf

Mark Scheme for Examiner

Introduction and General Advice

Introduces self (clean hands) ☐ ☐ ☐ ☐ ☐

Identifies patient (3 points of ID) ☐ ☐ ☐ ☐ ☐

Explains procedure, identifies concerns and obtains consent ☐ ☐ ☐ ☐ ☐

Checks chest X-ray and ultrasound scan ☐ ☐ ☐ ☐ ☐

Positions and exposes patient ☐ ☐ ☐ ☐ ☐

Identifies spot marked for pleural tap ☐ ☐ ☐ ☐ ☐

Percusses and auscultates to check location of effusion ☐ ☐ ☐ ☐ ☐

Preparation

Obtains equipment and checks expiry dates ☐ ☐ ☐ ☐ ☐

Washes hands, dons sterile gloves and single use apron ☐ ☐ ☐ ☐ ☐

Places drape over the patient ☐ ☐ ☐ ☐ ☐

Cleans site in a spiral pattern three times ☐ ☐ ☐ ☐ ☐

Performing the Pleural Tap

Injects local anesthetic using the 'withdraw and infiltrate' method ☐ ☐ ☐ ☐ ☐

Withdraws needle and syringe ☐ ☐ ☐ ☐ ☐

Inserts another needle and withdraws up to 50 mL of aspirate ☐ ☐ ☐ ☐ ☐

Applies pressure to insertion site and places dressing ☐ ☐ ☐ ☐ ☐

Finishing

Labels specimen bottles at the bedside ☐ ☐ ☐ ☐ ☐

Disposes of equipment ☐ ☐ ☐ ☐ ☐

Removes gloves and washes hands ☐ ☐ ☐ ☐ ☐

Documents procedure in the patient notes ☐ ☐ ☐ ☐ ☐

General Points

Talks throughout the procedure to the patient ☐ ☐ ☐ ☐ ☐

Disposes of all sharps immediately ☐ ☐ ☐ ☐ ☐

Avoids patient contamination (i.e. NTT) ☐ ☐ ☐ ☐ ☐

Questions and Answers for Candidate

What is the difference between pleural effusion and pulmonary oedema?

- A pleural effusion is fluid buildup in the space in between the parietal and visceral pleura of the lung. Pulmonary oedema is fluid leakage into the lung interstitium and alveoli

What are some common causes of an exudative pleural effusion?

- Malignancy
- Pulmonary embolism
- Pneumonia
- TB

Additional Questions to Consider

1. What are Light's criteria and when might they be used?
2. What further investigations might you order on the pleural fluid if malignancy is suspected?
3. How would you manage a small effusion secondary to a pneumonia?

Station 6: CHEST DRAIN

Mr Lodger is a 58-year-old man who has been in ITU following admission to hospital for severe community acquired pneumonia. The respiratory examination demonstrates decreased air entry and stony-dull percussion on the left side. A significant left-sided pleural effusion is confirmed on ultrasound and the decision is made to drain this collection via pleurocentesis. Please insert a chest drain.

Objectives

- Insert a thoracic chest drain
- Connect the drain correctly to the chest drain bottle
- Understand the principles of how to assess a correctly functioning chest drain

General Advice

- Obtain valid consent
- Inspect the chest X-ray and USS to detect the size and site of the pleural effusion
- Remember to adjust the position of the chest drain with regards to drainage of either pleural fluid or pneumothorax
- Always keep sight of the guidewire when using the Seldinger technique. One hand should always ensure that an adequate length of wire is available outside the patient
- Do not force the dilators or chest drain tube as this may lead to kinking of the guide wire and create false passages
- Check the patient's blood results before doing the procedure, particularly the platelet count and clotting function. Bloods for albumin, protein, LDH, and glucose are helpful in interpreting pleural fluid tests
- If the patient feels faint during the procedure, stop and withdraw the needle immediately and lie the patient down
- We have shown the procedure for drain insertion using a typical seldinger kit, but the choice of tube/method should always be considered (e.g. wide-bore tubes should always be used in preference to seldinger tubes in trauma where it is felt the latter would provide inadequate drainage of blood)

Equipment Checklist

(remember to check expiry dates on all equipment)

a) An assistant
b) Water-tight universal drain container with sterile tubing and connector
c) Sterile water
d) Chest drainage catheter equipment
   - Introducer needle
   - Guidewire
   - Dilators
   - Chest drain
   - 4-way tap
   - Male connector
e) Single use apron and sterile gloves
f) Chlorhexidine swab and spray
g) Suture pack and suture
h) Scalpel
i) 10 mL syringe, 25- gauge and 2 x 21- gauge needle (for LA)
j) 10 mL lidocaine 1%
k) Sterile pack with sterile towels and drape
l) Sharps bin
m) Sterile trolley
n) Sterile dressing

MEDICINE AND SURGERY

Explaining a Chest Drain to the Patient

1. A chest drain is a plastic tube, which allows us to drain fluid or air from the space, which has built up between your lungs and ribs

2. LA is injected around the area of skin where the needle is inserted to numb the skin and provide some pain relief

3. A guidewire is inserted through a needle in the skin, and into the space between your ribs and lung

4. The entry site is then widened and a plastic tube is inserted through the guide wire so that it is in the correct place

5. The other side of the plastic tube is connected to a plastic container with water inside that will allow any fluid or air to be drained

6. The plastic tube is secured with stitches and a dressing is put over the insertion area

7. We will need to obtain chest X-rays afterwards to check the drain is in the right position

Inserting a Chest Drain

Preparation

1. Introduce yourself to the patient and obtain written consent

2. Arrange all the equipment on a sterile trolley ready to be opened

3. Assemble the underwater seal by filling the universal chest drain container with an adequate amount of sterile water. Position the container near your assistant and the sterile tubing on the sterile trolley

4. Expose the patient from head to waist and position the patient sitting slightly rotated upright on the bed, with pillows cascaded below the shoulder and upper back

5. Spray the patient adequately with chlorhexidine spray down the mid-axillary line, plus front and back around the safe triangle. Leave to air dry (Fig 5.14)

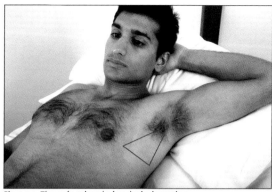

Fig 5.14: The safe triangle for drain insertion

'The 'safe triangle' is bordered by the:

• lateral border of the pectoralis major

• anterior border of the latissimus dorsi

• superiorly by the apex below the axilla

• inferiorly by the line at horizontal level of the nipple'

'Adequate draping helps to eliminate the passage of microorganisms between sterile and non-sterile and surfaces. Therefore, any unsterile surfaces (e.g. tubes, patient clothing) should be covered by the drape and not be visible or accessible during the remainder of the aseptic procedure'

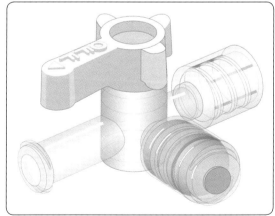

Fig 5.15: Correct position of the tap to prevent air entering the chest

Insertion

1. Scrub up aseptically and put on apron and sterile gloves

2. Open the sterile pack and arrange all equipment into the sterile field using an aseptic technique

3. Attach the chest drain to the 4-way tap and male connector and turn the rotator on the tap to prevent any air entering the drain (Fig 5.15)

4. Attach the 21-gauge needle to the 10mL syringe and draw up 5-10mL of lidocaine 1%

5. Clean the skin with chlorhexidine swabs in a spiral pattern three times

6. Drape the patient in a 'box' fashion with a clear view of the 'safe triangle' (Fig 5.16)

7. Determine the 4th or 5th intercostal space in the 'safe triangle'

8. Infiltrate the proposed area for drain insertion with LA. Use the 25-gauge to superficially anaesthetize the skin. Swap the 25-gauge with the second 21-gauge needle and anaesthetize down to the pleura, using the 'infiltrate and aspirate' method. Keep note of the depth of the needle when pleural fluid is aspirated

9. Withdraw the needle and dispose in sharps bin

10. Swap the 21-gauge with the introducer needle (now attached to the syringe) and re-determine the rib just below the intercostal space you intend to enter

11. Insert the introducer needle aiming to hit the upper border of the rib just palpated (Fig 5.17)

12. Aim into the intercostal space just above the upper border of the rib

13. Stop advancing when pleural fluid or air is aspirated. This should be a similar depth to that noted previously

14. If no pleural fluid or free air is aspirated, do not continue with the chest tube without further imaging guidance

15. Stabilise the introducer needle against the skin with your non-dominant hand to ensure that it remains immobile from this position

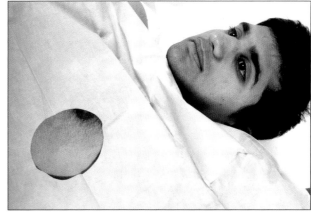

Fig 5.16: Draping the patient with adequate clearance

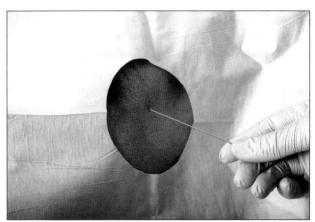

Fig 5.17: Correct positioning for introducer needle

The chest drain is typically in a looped shape and therefore can be angled either up or down depending on the substance being drained. Aim the chest drain upwards to drain air (in the case of a pneumothorax) or downwards to drain fluid (in the case of a pleural effusion)

MEDICINE AND SURGERY

'All needles should be inserted perpendicular to the skin, directly above the upper edge of the corresponding rib, into the pleural space occupied by the pleural fluid. This minimizes risk of the needle damaging the neurovascular bundle, which runs along the underside of the rib'

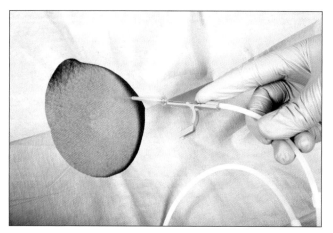

Fig 5.18: Removing the plastic sheath from the guidewire

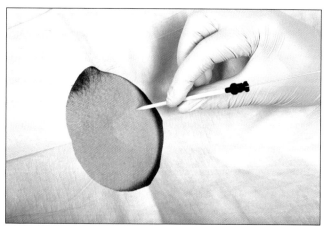

Fig 5.19: Correct positioning for dilators. The dilator should be inserted perpendicular to the skin following the same tract as the needle and guidewire previously

Insertion of the Chest Drain using the Seldinger Technique

1. Pick up the guidewire with your dominant hand and with your thumb pull back on the guidewire so the curved tip is now barely visible past the plastic cover. This is to straighten the tip of the guidewire

2. Detach the syringe from introducer. Insert the plastic top of the guidewire into the opening of the introducer needle and feed the guidewire into the pleural space with your thumb

3. Remove the plastic sheath from the guidewire when approximately 10cm remains and grab the guidewire with your non-dominant hand (Fig 5.18)

4. Remove the introducer needle from the skin by pulling it out over the guidewire and place it on the sterile tray with your dominant hand

5. Withdraw and re-insert the guidewire slightly to ensure that it moves freely

6. Make a small horizontal and vertical incision at the insertion point of the guidewire with the tip of the scalpel

7. Set the maximum penetration depth of the dilators using the depth previously noted during insertion of the introducer needle

8. Securing the guidewire's tip gently with your non-dominant hand, thread the first dilator through the guidewire until its set depth (Fig 5.19)

9. Repeat this process with the other dilators of increasing diameter

10. Remove the last dilator and secure the guidewire's tip gently with your non-dominant hand

11. Ensure that the tap at the end of the chest drain is closed to the outside environment to prevent air from entering the pleural cavity

12. Insert the chest drain over the guidewire perpendicular to the skin

Guidewires

- Always ensure that the guidewire is visible and secured with enough length outside the patient's body to prevent it being lost inside the patient

- A common pitfall is to kink the guidewire during insertion of dilators. A free moving guidewire indicates the absence of kinking and false passages through which the chest drain could be inserted

MEDICINE AND SURGERY

Securing the Chest Drain (5.20)

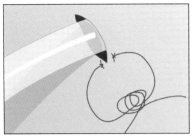

STEP 1: Enter the skin superficially, lateral to the chest tube on one side at its lower border with the suture, and exit the skin just above the entrance site at the upper border of the chest tube on the same side

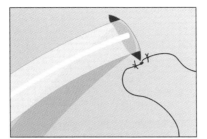

STEP 2: Pull the suture through the wound so there is an equal amount of string on both sides and tie a reef knot. Cut the needle from the suture and lay it on the sterile table for disposal later

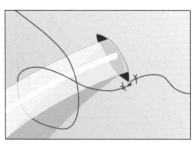

STEP 3: Loop the string from the lower border around the chest drain several times

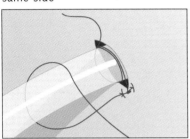

STEP 4: Loop the string from the upper border around the chest drain several times. The two ends should remain on opposite sides afterwards

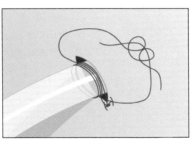

STEP 5: Tie another reef knot

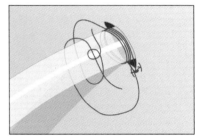

STEP 6: Wrap the remaining strings around the tube and tie another reef knot

Tying a Reef Knot (5.21)

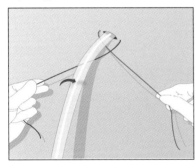

STEP 1: Hold the suture ends (RED in left hand, BLUE in right hand), ensuring the suture is wrapped around the back of the chest drain tubing

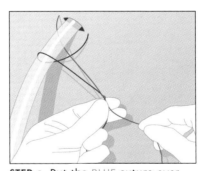

STEP 2: Put the BLUE suture over the top of the RED suture and hold the point where they meet with your left hand

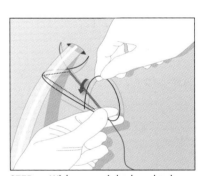

STEP 3: With your right hand take the RED suture end. Lift it up in the air, and then bring it down from above through the triangle formed by the sutures being crossed over

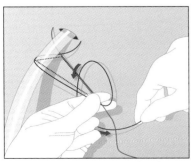

STEP 4: After going vertically down through the triangle, bring the RED suture end out from the underside of the triangle, to the right

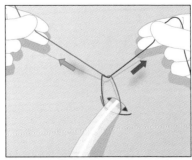

STEP 5: Pull the two suture ends. The sutures should lie at against the skin

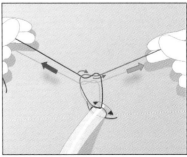

STEP 6: Repeat the steps above to form a sitting reef knot

Completing the Procedure

1. Apply two dressings in a 'duck bill' fashion above and below the chest drain
2. Connect the male end of the chest drain to the sterile tubing whilst ensuring that the chest drain does not dislodge from the patient
3. Ask your assistant to open the watertight universal drain container and present it to you
4. Place the rigid part of the sterile tubing through the opening. Ensure you remain sterile throughout this part of the procedure and that the chest drain does not dislodge from the patient (Fig 5.22)
5. Ensure that the rigid sterile tubing is well immersed in the sterile water but not obstructed by the bottom of the container
6. Check that the chest tube is draining the pleural effusion or bubbling is seen underwater in the sterile container
7. Remove the sterile drapes and dispose of any sharps
8. Order a post-procedure chest X-ray to review the position of the chest drain

Documenting the Procedure

Document under the following headings:
- Chest drain inserted
- Indications for the procedure
- Patient consent
- Relevant laboratory investigations (e.g. clotting, platelet count)
- Procedure technique, sterile preparation, anaesthetic use, amount of fluid obtained, appearance of fluid obtained, estimated blood loss
- Complications
- Subsequent tests ordered, if any (e.g. CXR/CT/USS)

> 'Rotate the wrist during insertion of the suture through the skin. This will ensure that the suture passes through the superficial layers of the skin, thereby minimising damage to internal structures and vasculature'

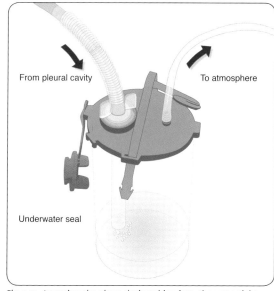

Fig 5.22: Inserting the chest drain tubing into the watertight drain container held by the assistant

Indications for performing a chest drain (BTS guidelines 2003)

Pneumothorax	Others
• In any ventilated patient	• Malignant pleural effusion
• Tension pneumothorax after initial needle relief	• Empyema and complicated parapneumonic pleural effusion
• Persistent or recurrent pneumothorax after simple aspiration	• Traumatic haemopneumothroax
• Large secondary spontaneous pneumothorax in patients age >50	• Postoperative – after thoracotomy, oesophagectomy or cardiac surgery (usually performed at the time of surgery)

Guideline:

BTS guidelines for the insertion of a chest drain, Thorax 2003 http://thorax.bmj.com/content/58/suppl_2/ii53.full#ref-7Thorax 2003;58:ii53-ii59 doi:10.1136/thorax.58.suppl_2.ii53

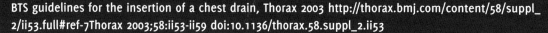

MEDICINE AND SURGERY

Mark Scheme for Examiner

Introduction and General Advice

Introduces self (clean hands)

Identifies patient (3 points of ID)

Explains procedure, identifies concerns and obtains consent

Checks chest X-ray and ultrasound scan, clotting and platelet count

Positions and exposes patient

Describes safe triangle and sprays with chlorhexidine

Preparation

Obtains equipment and checks expiry dates

Washes hands, puts on apron and sterile gloves

Sets up equipment in a logical fashion within hand reach

Adequately drapes patient

Cleans site in a spiral pattern three times

Inserting the Chest Drain

Identifies 4th/5th intercostal space in the safe triangle

Injects local anesthetic using the 'aspirate and infiltrate' method

Inserts introducer needle

Withdraws straw coloured aspirate or free air during deep infiltration

Secures introducer needle and removes syringe

Inserts the guidewire and keeps it secure. Removes introducer

Appropriately dilates and blunt dissects the insertion point

Rechecks that tap at the end of the chest drain is closed to air

Inserts chest drain over guidewire

Closes the wound and sutures the chest drain securely

Attaches the chest drain to the drain container
and checks for bubbling/aspiration of pleural fluid

Finishing

Disposes of equipment

Removes drapes, gloves and washes hands

Documents procedure in the patient notes

Orders post procedure chest X-ray

General Points

Talks throughout the procedure to the patient

Disposes of all sharps immediately

Avoids patient contamination (i.e. NTT)

MEDICINE AND SURGERY

Questions and Answers for Candidate

Are abnormal blood clotting or platelet counts contraindications for insertion of a chest drain?

- There is no evidence currently that demonstrates bleeding complications of chest drain insertions due to abnormal clotting or platelet counts. However these should be corrected where possible as good practice

Additional Questions to Consider

1. Why should the chest drain tube be attached to an underwater seal?
2. Why is the 'safe triangle' recommended for chest drain insertion?
3. When administering LA, why do we aspirate prior to infiltration?

Station 7: DIAGNOSTIC ASCITIC TAP

Mr Brody is a 48-year-old man who presents to his GP with difficulty breathing, abdominal distension and cachexia. A long-standing history of alcohol abuse is discovered along with shifting dullness and a fluid thrill. Subsequent investigations demonstrate a cirrhotic liver and gross abdominal ascites. Please perform a diagnostic aspiration of the ascites and interpret your findings.

Objectives

- Perform a diagnostic ascitic tap
- Interpret the results

General Advice

- Obtain valid consent

- Ultrasound guidance is recommended to mark the ideal location for an ascitic tap. This ensures that the procedure can be performed as successfully and safely as possible. The following information may also be helpful and ideally should be requested from the sonographer prior to the procedure:

  o   Distance from skin to fluid (in cm)

  o   Distance from skin to the midpoint of the collection

- An abdominal ultrasound scan will also provide information about the likely underlying aetiology including the presence of lymphadenopathy, splenomegaly and portal hypertension

- Ensure that the patient has passed urine prior to the procedure

- Ensure that you have undertaken a full history and examination on the patient, making note of any clotting disorders. Prior to starting the procedure make sure you have checked the results of the patient's recent clotting screen and platelet count. At the time of ascitic tap, perform venepuncture. Check serum protein, albumin, U&Es, glucose, LDH (to help determine if transudate or exudate) plus any additional tests that may be considered

Equipment Checklist

(remember to check expiry dates on all equipment)

a) Sterile gloves and single use apron
b) 3 x chlorhexidine swabs
c) 21-gauge needle
d) 50 mL syringe (for ascitic aspirate)
e) Sterile pack with sterile towels and drape
f) Sterile universal container
g) Sterile gauze and dressing
h) Sharps bin

Explaining a Diagnostic Ascitic Tap to the Patient

1. An ascitic tap is a procedure which allows us to obtain a sample of fluid present inside your tummy
2. You may have to have an ultrasound scan of your abdomen before the procedure and the radiologist will mark the spot where we take the sample from
3. The sample is then obtained by inserting a needle through the skin, into the space between your abdominal organs where the fluid has leaked
4. The fluid obtained is then sent to the laboratory for testing
5. The needle is then removed and a dressing put over that area
6. Although unlikely, it may not be possible to obtain a sample of fluid

Performing an Ascitic Tap

Preparation

1. Introduce yourself to the patient and obtain written consent
2. Gather your equipment
3. Expose the patient's abdomen
4. Position the patient supine on the bed with their hands under their head
5. Percuss the area around the spot marked for the ascitic tap, ensuring that the marked spot corresponds with dullness
6. Open the sterile pack and arrange all equipment into the sterile field using an aseptic technique

Aseptic Technique

1. Wash hands and don sterile gloves and single use apron
2. Apply sterile drapes. Clean the insertion area in a spiral pattern three times, using chlorhexidine swabs (Fig 5.23)
3. Place all equipment in the sterile field
4. Attach the 21-gauge needle to a 50mL syringe for ascitic aspiration
5. Advance the 21-gauge needle and 50mL syringe into the abdomen until ascitic fluid is aspirated and draw up to 50mL of ascitic fluid (Fig 5.24)
6. Withdraw the needle and place into the sterile field
7. Apply pressure with sterile gauze and then cover with a sterile dressing if required
8. Transfer aspirate into sterile universal container and send to the laboratory for:
   - Albumin, protein, LDH, glucose
   - Absolute white cell count (WCC)
9. If indicated, consider sending the sample for:
   - Cytology (if underlying malignancy is suspected)
   - Acid-fast staining (for tuberculosis)

Documenting the Procedure

Document under the following headings:
- Ascitic tap performed on patient
- Indications for the procedure
- Patient consent
- Relevant laboratory investigations (e.g. INR/PTT, platelet count)
- Procedure technique, sterile preparation, amount of fluid obtained, appearance of fluid obtained
- Complications
- Tests ordered (e.g. USS)

'If USS guidance is not available, the insertion site for an ascitic tap is approximately 15cm laterally to the umbilicus usually in either the right or left lower abdominal quadrant. It is also possible to insert 2cm below the umbilicus in the midline, through the linea alba. Avoid areas of prominent superficial veins (caput medusae), scars and palpable masses'

'Although an ascitic tap is not contraindicated in patients with abnormal clotting profiles, it would be advisable to give pooled platelets in severe thrombocytopaenia (platelets <40,000 per microlitre of blood)'

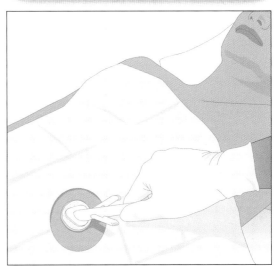

Fig 5.23: This is a sterile procedure so careful preparation is required

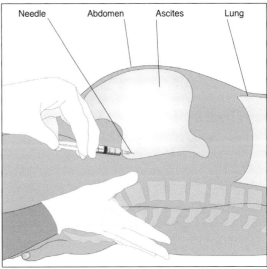

Fig 5.24: The correct position for an ascitic tap procedure, ensure you have percussed the abdomen prior to the procedure

MEDICINE AND SURGERY

Mark Scheme for Examiner

Introduction and General Advice

Introduces self (clean hands) ☐ ☐ ☐ ☐ ☐

Identifies patient (3 points of ID) ☐ ☐ ☐ ☐ ☐

Explains procedure, identifies concerns and obtains consent ☐ ☐ ☐ ☐ ☐

Positions and exposes patient ☐ ☐ ☐ ☐ ☐

Checks ultrasound scan and clotting ☐ ☐ ☐ ☐ ☐

Identifies spot marked ascitic tap, percusses to check ☐ ☐ ☐ ☐ ☐

Preparation

Obtains equipment and checks expiry dates ☐ ☐ ☐ ☐ ☐

Washes hands, dons apron and sterile gloves ☐ ☐ ☐ ☐ ☐

Places drape over patient ☐ ☐ ☐ ☐ ☐

Cleans site in a spiral pattern three times ☐ ☐ ☐ ☐ ☐

Performing the Ascitic Tap

Inserts needle and withdraws up to 50mL of aspirate ☐ ☐ ☐ ☐ ☐

Applies pressure to insertion site and place dressing ☐ ☐ ☐ ☐ ☐

Finishing

Labels specimen bottles at the bedside ☐ ☐ ☐ ☐ ☐

Disposes of equipment ☐ ☐ ☐ ☐ ☐

Removes gloves/apron and washes hands ☐ ☐ ☐ ☐ ☐

Documents procedure in the patient notes ☐ ☐ ☐ ☐ ☐

General Points

Talks throughout the procedure to the patient ☐ ☐ ☐ ☐ ☐

Disposes of all sharps immediately ☐ ☐ ☐ ☐ ☐

Avoids patient contamination (i.e. NTT) ☐ ☐ ☐ ☐ ☐

What should you always suspect if a patient becomes unwell after an ascitic tap?

- Spontaneous bacterial peritonitis

What are the different grades of ascites?

- Grade 1 = only detectable by USS
- Grade 2 = detected by moderate abdominal distension
- Grade 3 = detected by marked abdominal distension

Additional Questions to Consider

1. How is the serum-ascites albumin gradient (SAAG) calculated?
2. What does a SAAG of >11 g/l signify?
3. What are the causes of a transudative ascites?
4. What ascitic WCC is diagnostic of SBP?
5. What is the treatment of SBP?

Station 8: THERAPEUTIC PARACENTESIS

Mrs Walker is a 64-year-old alcoholic woman with large volume ascites refractory to diuretic therapy. She is complaining of increasing abdominal pain and shortness of breath. Perform a therapeutic ascitic drain to alleviate her symptoms.

Objectives

- Perform a therapeutic ascitic drain

General Advice

- Obtain valid consent

- Ultrasound guidance is recommended to mark the ideal location for an ascitic tap. This ensures that the procedure can be performed as successfully and safely as possible. The following information may also be helpful and ideally should be requested from the sonographer prior to the procedure:

  o Distance from skin to fluid (in cm)

  o Distance from the skin to the midpoint of the collection

- Ensure that the patient has passed urine prior to the procedure

- Ensure the patient has adequate IV access to give albumin if needed

- Ensure that you have undertaken a full history and examination on the patient, making note of any clotting disorders. Prior to starting the procedure make sure you have checked the results of the patient's recent clotting screen and platelet count

Equipment Checklist

(remember to check expiry dates on all equipment)
(Fig 5.25)

a) Sterile gloves and single use apron
b) Sterile drape
c) 3 x chlorhexidine swabs
d) 25-gauge needle
e) 2 x 21-gauge needles
f) 10 mL syringe (for LA)
g) 10 mL lidocaine 1%
h) Bonanno catheter and trocar (introducer)
i) Scalpel (optional)
j) 3 x IV cannula dressings to fix ascitic drain to skin
k) 2L catheter bag, and connector tube

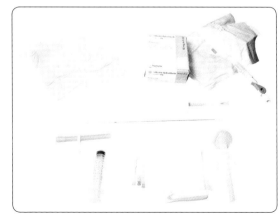

Fig 5.25: Equipment required to perform an abdominal paracentesis

Explaining an Abdominal Paracentesis to the Patient

1. An ascitic drain is a plastic tube that we place through the skin of your belly to allow us to drain away the excess fluid that has accumulated inside

2. You may have an ultrasound scan of your belly before the procedure and the radiologist will mark the spot where we take the sample from

3. An IV line will be placed into your arm and some blood will also be taken before the procedure

4. LA is injected around the area of skin where the needle is inserted to numb the skin and provide some pain relief

5. You may need some fluid via a drip depending on the amount of fluid drained

6. The drain will be removed after six hours

Performing an Abdominal Paracentesis

Preparation

1. Introduce yourself to the patient and obtain consent

2. Cannulate the patient

3. Obtain the equipment and a clean trolley

4. Expose the patient's abdomen and ask the patient to keep their hands under their head

5. Position the patient supine on the bed

6. Percuss the abdomen and identify the presence of ascites as suggested by shifting dullness. If you are not confident that there is a significant volume of ascites, do not proceed until a point has been marked with ultrasound assistance

7. Open the sterile pack and arrange all equipment into the sterile field using an aseptic technique

8. Clamp the connector tube (Fig 5.26)

Aseptic Technique

1. Wash hands and don sterile gloves and single use apron

2. Apply sterile drapes

3. Attach the 21-gauge needle to the 10 mL syringe and aspirate 5-10 mL of 1% lidocaine

4. Mark the site and clean the area in a spiral pattern three times (Fig 5.27)

5. Inject LA; use 25-gauge needle to superficially anaesthetise the skin

6. Swap the 25-gauge with another 21-gauge needle and alternately aspirate whilst infiltrating LA down towards the peritoneum

7. Withdraw the LA needle when straw coloured fluid is easily aspirated and note the depth of the needle

8. Prepare the Bonanno catheter by sliding the outer plastic sheath over the catheter to straighten the curved tip (Fig 5.28 and 5.29)

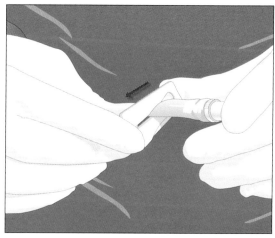

Fig 5.26: Prepare your equipment

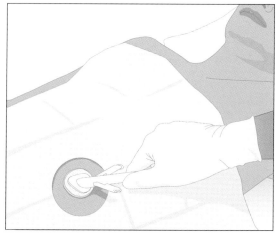

Fig 5.27: Ensure the abdomen is sterilised for this procedure

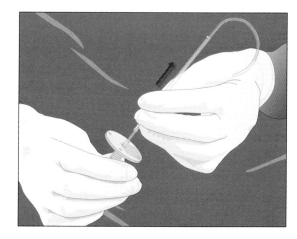

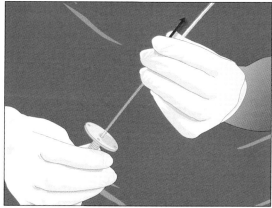

Fig 5.28 (top) and 5.29 (bottom): First, straighten the tip by slowly sliding the plastic sheath upwards

MEDICINE AND SURGERY

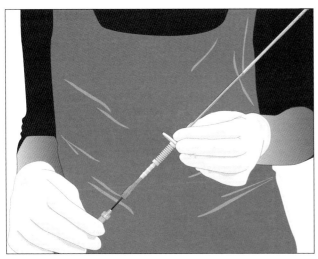

Fig 5.30: Insert the metal trocar

9. Insert the metal trocar inside the catheter and secure it to the catheter base (Fig 5.30)

10. Completely remove the outer plastic sheath

11. Carefully push the catheter into the anaesthetized area, keeping full control of the needle at the point of contact at the skin (Fig 5.31)

12. If excessive force is required to puncture the skin, use the scalpel to make a small incision in the skin to allow the catheter to pass more freely

13. Continue to advance the catheter into the peritoneal cavity until ascitic fluid can be seen draining back along the needle

14. Advance the needle a further centimetre to ensure the tip of the plastic catheter is within the peritoneal cavity

15. Unscrew the trocar from the catheter and advance the catheter over the trocar without moving the trocar any further

16. Once the catheter is fully inserted, remove the metal trocar (Fig 5.32). The plastic tube remains in situ (Fig 5.33)

17. Attach the clamped rubber connector tube to the catheter (Fig 5.34)

18. Connect the catheter bag and place it below the patient (Fig 5.35)

19. Secure the catheter to the skin using the IV cannula dressings

20. Unclamp the connector tube and ensure the ascites is draining well and note the colour of the fluid being drained

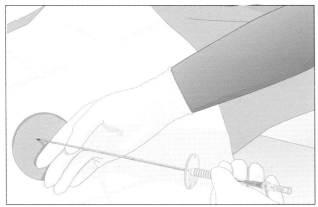

Fig 5.31: Ensure you have full control over the catheter when inserting

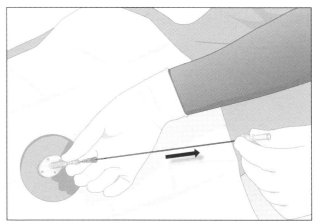

Fig 5.32: After advancing the catheter, gently remove the trocar

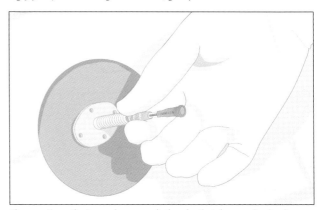

Fig 5.33: Once the trocar is removed, the plastic tube remains in situ

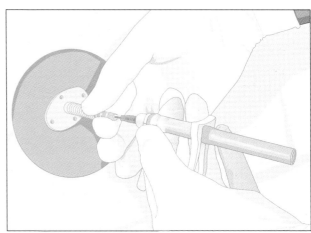

Fig 5.34: Attach the connecting tubing

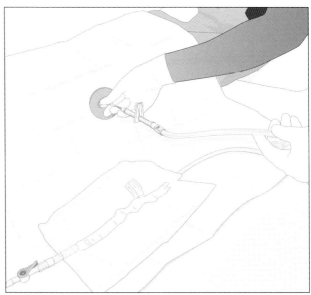

Fig 5.35: Connect the catheter bag

MEDICINE AND SURGERY

Documenting the Procedure

Document under the following headings:

- Ascitic drain performed on patient
- Indications for the procedure
- Patient consent
- Relevant laboratory investigations (e.g. INR/PTT, platelet count)
- Procedure technique, sterile preparation, anaesthetic and amount used, appearance of fluid obtained
- Complications
- Time the drain should be removed (usually 6-12 hours after insertion)
- Prescribe 100 mL of 20% human albumin solution for every 2-3 L of ascitic fluid drained (depending on local guidelines)

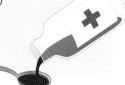

Causes of ascites:
- Liver cirrhosis (75%)
- Malignancy (10%)
- Heart failure (3%)
- TB (2%)

Complications of an Ascitic Drain

Common (>1%)	Rare (<0.1%)
Failure to collect fluid	Haemoperitoneum
Persistent leak from the puncture site	Bowel perforation
Wound infection	Death (due to bleeding or infection)
Abdominal wall haematoma	Haemoperitoneum

Guideline:

Guidelines on the management of ascites, British Society of Gastroenterology, 2006
http://www.bsg.org.uk/clinical-guidelines/liver/guidelines-on-the-management-of-ascites-in-cirrhosis.html

Mark Scheme for Examiner

Introduction and General Advice

Introduces self (clean hands) ☐ ☐ ☐ ☐ ☐

Identifies patient (3 points of ID) ☐ ☐ ☐ ☐ ☐

Explains procedure, identifies concerns and obtains consent ☐ ☐ ☐ ☐ ☐

Positions and exposes patient ☐ ☐ ☐ ☐ ☐

Checks ultrasound scan and clotting ☐ ☐ ☐ ☐ ☐

Identifies spot marked for ascitic drain, percusses to check ☐ ☐ ☐ ☐ ☐

Preparation

Obtains/prepares equipment (including clamping connector tubing) and checks all expiry dates ☐ ☐ ☐ ☐ ☐

Washes hands, dons sterile gloves and apron ☐ ☐ ☐ ☐ ☐

Places drape over patient ☐ ☐ ☐ ☐ ☐

Cleans site in a spiral pattern three times ☐ ☐ ☐ ☐ ☐

Inserting the Asictic Drain

Injects local anesthetic using the 'withdraw and infiltrate' method

□ □ □ □ □

Withdraws straw coloured aspirate during deep infiltration

□ □ □ □ □

Withdraws needle and syringe

□ □ □ □ □

Pushes catheter into anaesthetised area, until fluid seen, and then advances a further centimeter

□ □ □ □ □

Advances catheter over trocar

□ □ □ □ □

Removes trocar and attaches catheter to the rubber connector tube

□ □ □ □ □

Secures Bonnano catheter to skin and connects to a catheter bag (unclamping the connector tube)

□ □ □ □ □

Finishing

Disposes of equipment

□ □ □ □ □

Removes gloves/apron and washes hands

□ □ □ □ □

Documents procedure in the patient notes

□ □ □ □ □

General Points

Talks throughout the procedure to the patient

□ □ □ □ □

Disposes of all sharps immediately

□ □ □ □ □

Avoids patient contamination (i.e. NTT)

□ □ □ □ □

Questions and Answers for Candidate

What is refractory ascites?

- Ascites that fails to respond to intense diuretic therapy or ascites that occurs in a patient in whom intense diuretic therapy is not tolerated

Additional Questions to Consider

1. What proportion of patients with liver cirrhosis develop ascites? What is the associated mortality over the next few years?

2. What medical strategies are employed in the treatment of ascites?

3. What is the role of dietary salt restriction in the management of ascites?

4. What is TIPS and what are the risks and benefits of this procedure?

Station 9: LUMBAR PUNCTURE

Mr Waters is a 22-year-old university student who presents to the Emergency Department with an acute severe headache. Associated symptoms include fever, vomiting and photophobia. On examination you note marked neck stiffness and Kernig's sign is positive. There are no features suggestive of raised intracranial pressure. You strongly suspect bacterial meningitis and after a CT scan is performed, you are asked by your registrar to perform a LP in order to confirm the diagnosis.

Objectives

- Perform a LP
- Interpret the results

General Advice

- Performing a LP allows the clinician to obtain a sample of cerebrospinal fluid (CSF) from the subarachnoid space below the level at which the spinal cord terminates (L1/L2)
- As a junior doctor you should only perform this procedure following adequate instruction and under close supervision
- The key contraindication to performing a LP is raised intracranial pressure (ICP) – the combination of which may result in tonsillar herniation (i.e. 'coning')
- A head CT scan is generally performed prior to performing an LP

Equipment Checklist

(remember to check expiry dates on all equipment) (Fig 5.36)

a) Sterile gloves and single use apron
b) Chlorhexidine swabs
c) Procedure tray with sterile drape and swabs
d) Sterile dressing
e) 10 mL syringe
f) 10 mL lidocaine 1%
g) 25-gauge needle
h) 2 x 21-gauge needles
i) LP kit:
   - LP needle (typically 22-gauge)
   - 3-way tap
   - Manometer
   - CSF collection tubes (for microbiology and biochemistry including glucose)

Explaining an LP to the Patient

1. An LP is a procedure used to obtain a sample of cerebrospinal fluid – a type of body fluid which bathes the brain and spinal cord
2. It is important to obtain a sample where possible, because analysis of this fluid allows the medical team to ensure the correct diagnosis is made and appropriate treatment given
3. You will be asked to lie on the bed on your left hand side with your knees drawn up to your chest and lower back exposed
4. A needle is inserted into the lower part of the spine where the spinal cord ends, thereby reducing the risk of damage to the cord
5. An injection of local anaesthetic will be administered first into the skin overlying the puncture site in order to reduce pain; however, you may still experience a sensation of pressure/discomfort
6. A special needle will then be inserted into the space containing the cerebrospinal fluid and samples of the fluid will be taken
7. You may experience a headache and nausea following the procedure – this is the most common side effect. You will also need to lie flat for an hour after the procedure

Contraindications to performing an LP:
- Raised ICP
- Coagulopathy or low platelet count
- Cutaneous infection at the LP site

Features suggestive of raised ICP or intracerebral mass:
- Papilloedema
- Focal neurological signs
- Decreased level of consciousness (GCS <8/15)
- Bradycardia, hypertension and an irregular breathing pattern (Cushing's triad)

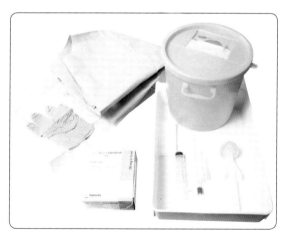

Fig 5.36: Not all wards will have the equipment for this procedure. Ensure you are aware where you can obtain all the equipment you need

Performing a LP

1. Introduce yourself, check the patient's ID and obtain informed consent
2. Ask the patient to adopt the left lateral position with their lumbar spine exposed
3. Position the patient with maximum flexion of the spine, hips and knees (widening the intervertebral space)
4. Palpate the superior iliac crest and then follow a vertical line down to the space between the vertebral spines immediately below (corresponds to L3/L4 or L4/L5 intervertebral disc space)
5. Mark this space with an indentation/pen
6. Wash hands. Put on sterile gloves and single use apron. Drape the lumbar spine region
7. Check all of the equipment and open onto the procedure tray
8. Sterilize the skin using the swabs
9. Attach the 21-gauge needle to the 10 mL syringe and draw up the lidocaine
10. Infiltrate the lidocaine superficially at the marked location, using a 25-gauge needle
11. Exchange the 25-gauge needle for the larger 21-gauge needle and continue to infiltrate lidocaine into the deeper tissues (N.B. ensure you aspirate before injecting to reduce the risk of accidental intravascular injection)
12. Wait approximately one minute for the LA to take effect
13. Take the LP needle and introduce it into the skin at the marked site, with the bevel of the needle pointing up (Fig 5.37)
14. Carefully advance the needle through the spinal ligaments, feeling a 'give' in resistance as you penetrate the dura mater and enter the subarachnoid space
15. Now withdraw the stylet from the LP needle and watch for CSF to begin dripping from the needle cuff
16. Attach the manometer and 3-way tap to the needle in a vertical position, allowing you to measure CSF pressure (wait for the fluid to stop rising up the column and read off the value)
17. Open the 3-way tap and allow 5-10 drops of CSF to drip into each of the three collection tubes (label these tubes 1 to 3 in the order of collection)
18. If still dripping, collect a glucose sample as well
19. Reinsert the stylet to stop the flow of CSF and remove the needle
20. Apply a sterile dressing

Finishing the Procedure

- Remove the drape and ensure safe disposal of sharps/packaging
- Prescribe simple analgesia PRN for any resultant headache
- Label the collection tubes appropriately and send to the lab for:
  o MC&S
  o Cell count
  o Biochemistry (protein and glucose)
- Document the procedure and any complications/technical difficulty
- To be able to interpret the results of a LP, a capillary blood sample is also necessary to allow measurement of plasma glucose levels

The anatomical layers that are penetrated when inserted a LP needle are (Fig 5.38):

1. Skin
2. Supraspinous ligament
3. Interspinous ligament and ligamentum flavum
4. (Extradural space)
5. Dura mater
6. Arachnoid mater

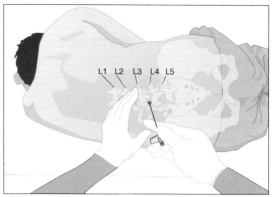

Fig 5.37: Take time to position the patient correctly before inserting the LP needle (drapes not shown)

L1 L2 L3 L4 L5

'When introducing the LP needle, imagine you are aiming for the umbilicus — this will help to ensure correct positioning. Many doctors will tell you that this practical skill involves a certain amount of "feel" — practice makes perfect!'

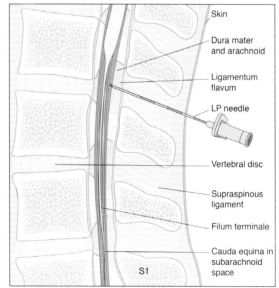

Skin

Dura mater and arachnoid

Ligamentum flavum

LP needle

Vertebral disc

Supraspinous ligament

Filum terminale

Cauda equina in subarachnoid space

S1

Fig 5.38: The key layers penetrated when inserting a LP needle

MEDICINE AND SURGERY

Endotracheal Tube: (Fig 5.43)

1. This is a 'cuffed endotracheal tube' and is an example of a definitive airway

2. This device is used in anaesthetics and in intensive care during the intubation and ventilation of unconscious patients

3. This device needs to be inserted by a trained health professional in a controlled environment. It is inserted into the trachea under direct vision with the use of a laryngoscope to identify the glottis. After insertion the balloon cuff is inflated with the use of a syringe to keep the tube in place and prevent aspiration of gastric contents into the respiratory tract

4. Tube complications include misplacement of the tube into the oesophagus and descent of the tube into a main bronchus (commonly right main bronchus). Also: impaction of the tube against the airway, dental/lip/gum trauma, pulmonary aspiration of gastric contents, oesophageal or tracheal perforation, subglottic stenosis, and vocal cord paralysis

5. A relative contraindication to intubation includes cervical spine injury, where immobilisation makes intubation difficult. In addition, in severe airway trauma or obstruction, an emergency cricothyrotomy is likely to be more useful

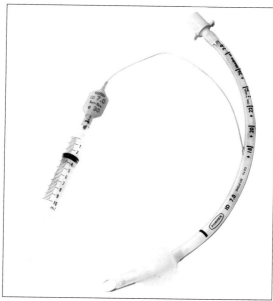

Fig 5.43: Endotracheal tube

NG Tube: (Fig 5.44)

1. This is a naso-gastric tube of which there are two types: fine and wide-bore

2. Fine-bore tubes are used for enteral feeding in patients with an unsafe swallow assessment on the ward, and also following gastrointestinal surgery. Wide-bore tubes are typically used to provide gastric decompression in patients with bowel obstruction or following elective upper gastrointestinal surgery

3. The distance required to insert the tube is sized by measuring the distance of the tube from the nostril to the xiphesternum passing via the tragus of the ear. The lower 10cm is then lubricated and advanced along the base of the nasal cavity in an upright patient. The patient is asked to sip water using a straw when the tube reaches the posterior pharynx. This manoeuvre aids the introduction of the tube into the oesophagus. The tube is inserted to the sized distance and then a little more to ensure correct positioning which is confirmed via testing aspirates with pH paper and chest X-ray

4. The most common complications are damage to the nasal turbinates (resulting in bleeding) during insertion and misplacement e.g. into the trachea

5. NG tubes are contraindicated in patients with base of skull fractures, severe mid-face trauma and recent nasal surgery. Relative contraindications include oesophageal varices, an obstructed oesophagus and coagulation abnormalities

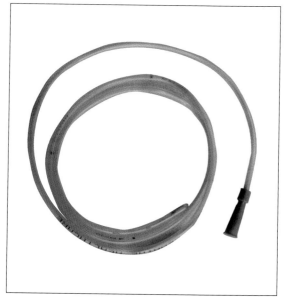

Fig 5.44: NG tube

Bag Valve Mask: (Fig 5.45)

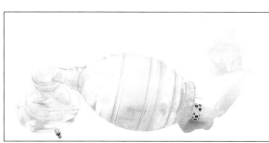

Fig 5.45: Bag valve mask

1. This is a bag valve mask used to provide positive pressure ventilation
2. This is used to oxygenate and ventilate patients who are not breathing or breathing inadequately. This device is frequently used in anaesthetics and in the acute care of patients until a more definitive airway is implemented
3. The bag valve mask can be connected to an oxygen port on the wall to provide concentrated oxygen but also works independently and is self filling. The mask is triangular in shape and its tip should be placed just over the bridge of the patient's nose. The larger portion of the mask should be placed between the lower lips and the chin to provide a good seal. Although one person can operate this device, it is more comfortable with two, where one person places the mask firmly on the patients face whilst simultaneously providing a jaw thrust, and the other squeezes the bag
4. Complications of a bag valve mask include aspiration, hypoventilation and hyperventilation; you must use with care in patients with suspected cervical-spine trauma or facial fractures
5. Bag mask valve ventilation is relatively contraindicated after paralysis and induction due to the increased risk of aspiration. An absolute contraindication to its use is in complete upper airway obstruction

Otoscope: (Fig 5.46)

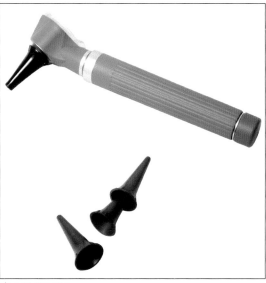

Fig 5.46: Otoscope

1. This device is an otoscope, and can be separated into four main types: direct, indirect, pneumatic and operating. The standard direct otoscope can either be wall mounted or battery operated. The device can additionally be attached to different sized speculums
2. It is used by doctors to examine the external auditory canal and tympanic membrane for outer and middle ear pathology
3. The direct otoscope is typically held in the same hand as the side of the ear being examined. It is held the same way as a pen, with the fingers placed on its neck next to the eyepiece and with the speculum facing away from the operator. After activating the light source and inspecting the external auditory canal and surrounding areas, the pinna is manually retracted superiorly and posteriorly with the other hand. The otoscope is gently introduced into the ear canal with the little finger extended and rested on the patient to provide stability to the instrument
4. Complications are rare but mainly include trauma to the ear canal

MEDICINE AND SURGERY

Common Instruments
Here is a list of other common equipment that will be useful to look up:

Lines:
Central venous line
Hickman line
Swan Ganz catheter

Colorectal:
Rigid sigmoidoscope
Flexible sigmoidoscope
Gabriel syringe
Laparoscopic ports

Orthopaedic:
Knee prostheses
Hip prostheses
Dynamic hip screw
Medullary nail

Fluids:
Crystalloids:
Hartmann's solution
Normal saline
Dextrose saline

Colloids:
Gelofusin
Albumin
Blood products

Airways:
Nasopharyngeal airway
Laryngeal mask airway
Tracheostomy tube

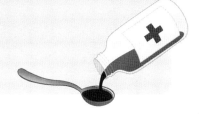

Mark Scheme for Examiner

Introduction

Identifies name of equipment ☐ ☐ ☐ ☐ ☐

Describes main indications for use ☐ ☐ ☐ ☐ ☐

Describes step-by-step instructions on safe use of device ☐ ☐ ☐ ☐ ☐

Outlines complications ☐ ☐ ☐ ☐ ☐

Outlines contraindications ☐ ☐ ☐ ☐ ☐

Practical Skills

Holds equipment in correct position ☐ ☐ ☐ ☐ ☐

Simulates use of equipment on manikin correctly ☐ ☐ ☐ ☐ ☐

General Points

Speaks clearly with a measured pace ☐ ☐ ☐ ☐ ☐

Demonstrates confidence with equipment use ☐ ☐ ☐ ☐ ☐

Answers questions on equipment ☐ ☐ ☐ ☐ ☐

Questions and Answers for Candidate

What device can be used to safely provide rescue breaths during CPR?

- A pocket face mask is often used and contains an attachable one way valve to protect the operator from infectious bodily fluids such as vomit

Where are the defibrillator pads placed on a person?

- One pad is placed over the left praecordium at the lower part of the chest and the second typically below the right clavicle. If the patient had a pacemaker you would place the pads at least 8 cm away

How many litres of oxygen do you connect to nasal cannulae?

- A nasal cannula is typically used to carry 2-4 litres per minute of oxygen to the patient. Using flow rates above five litres can cause discomfort to the patient as the flow becomes turbulent

What preliminary test can you do to check if the NG tube is in the right place without pH paper or a chest X-ray?

- Inject air into the NG tube and auscultate at the left costal angle. Passage of air will be heard as it enters the stomach if the NG tube is in the right place. Note: a chest X-ray may be ordered to definitively check for correct placement of an NG tube

Additional Questions to Consider

1. What is the difference between crystalloids and colloids, and what are their respective indications?

2. What are the typical daily fluid requirements for maintenance of the average adult who is nil-by-mouth?

3. When can a hard cervical collar be removed from a patient with suspected cervical-spine injury?

Station 12: SUTURING

Mr Harrison, aged 27 years, has presented to the emergency department with a wound to his forearm. Please suture the wound together using a simple technique.

Objectives

- To be able to perform basic suturing

General Advice

- Start this station by assessing the wound to see if it requires referral to senior or specialist surgical colleagues
- It is important to check the neurovascular supply to the region and involve senior staff where wounds involve tendons, nerves, or large vessels
- It may be useful to order an X-ray where retained or deep foreign bodies are suspected
- A plastic surgery referral is essential for complex facial lacerations, especially those involving the vermilion line (the border between the lips and skin)

Explaining Suturing to the Patient

1. Suturing is a technique used to close up wounds using a needle attached to thread
2. Before starting, the wound will be cleaned, and a numbing agent will be injected around the cut for pain relief
3. The wound will then be closed up with sutures and a bandage applied over the area
4. Your wound will be inspected at a later date and the sutures may be removed when the wound has healed
5. It is important to inform the doctor if the wound looks infected or continues to bleed considerably after discharge

Equipment Checklist

(remember to check expiry dates on all equipment)

a) Iodine solution
b) Sterile water
c) Gauze
d) Needle holder
e) Toothed forceps
f) Scissors
g) Suture(s): e.g. 4/0 synthetic, non-absorbable monofilament with a curved needle
h) Lidocaine with 1/200 000 adrenaline (to minimise bleeding, but dont use adrenaline on extremities due to vasoconstrictive effect)
i) 5 mL syringe and 21-gauge needle
j) 25-gauge needle to administer
k) Equipment trolley
l) Sharps bin
m) An assistant
n) Sterile gloves
o) Sterile dressing

Note: a lot of this equipment may come in a preformed 'sterile pack' for suturing

Suturing

Procedure Preparation

1. Obtain valid consent
2. Obtain equipment, wash hands and don gloves using the aseptic technique (Fig 5.47)
3. Assemble the suturing equipment on a sterile field on the equipment trolley
4. Withdraw lidocaine into 5 mL syringe via 21-gauge needle
5. Detach the needle without re-sheathing, and discard it in a sharps bin
6. Attach a 25-gauge needle with its sheath on and place the needle and syringe into the needle's packet

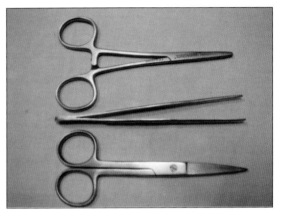

Fig 5.47: From top to bottom: needle holder; forceps and scissors

'It is important to inject LA before cleaning the wound with iodine soaked gauze'

Wound Preparation

1. Remove large visible debris from the wound using forceps
2. Use sterile water to soak gauze and clean the wound gently
3. Administer LA into the skin and soft tissues around the wound in a circular pattern via the 'aspirate and infiltrate' technique
4. Soak iodine solution on gauze and clean the wound
5. Dry the wound with a clean gauze

Suturing (basic interrupted suturing technique)

1. Hold the needle holder in your dominant hand with your thumb and ring finger (Fig 5.48)
2. Hold the toothed forceps in your other hand using a pen grip (Fig 5.49)
3. Remove the needle and suture from the packaging with the needle holder and reposition the needle using the forceps (Fig 5.50)
4. Bring your thumb and ring finger together to lock the needle into the needle holder, several clicks should be heard
5. The first suture should be in the centre of the wound
6. With the forceps, gently manipulate the wound's edge
7. Insert the needle perpendicular to the skin's surface approximately 5mm from the wound edge (Fig 5.51)
8. Advance the needle through the wound in a circular arc aiming to exit in the middle of the wound
9. Grasp the needle with the forceps taking care not to blunt the tip of the needle
10. Release the needle from the needle holder
11. Withdraw the needle with the forceps and re-grip with the needle holder
12. Use the forceps as a pulley to leave approximately 4cm of thread at the original insertion site
13. Re-insert the needle from within the wound and aim to exit about 5mm from the wound edge (Fig 5.52)
14. Once again, grasp the needle with the forceps, release from needle holder and withdraw the needle to pull the thread taut

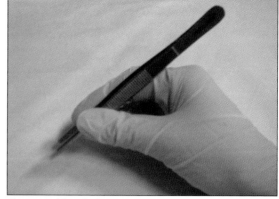

Fig 5.49: Holding the forceps

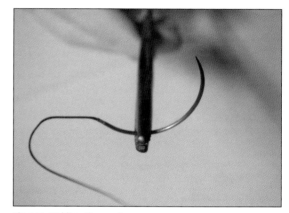

Fig 5.50: Holding the needle

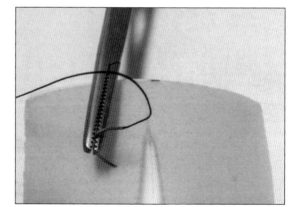

Fig 5.51: Inserting the needle

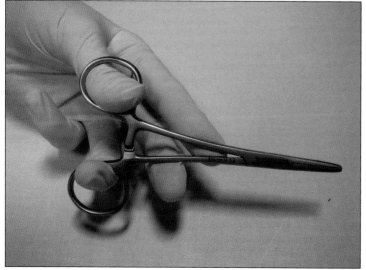

Fig 5.48: Holding the needle holder

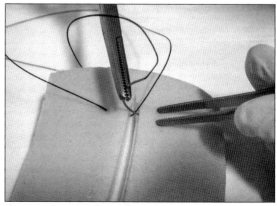

Fig 5.52: Reinserting the needle on the opposite side

Tying a Surgical Knot

1. Place the needle holder in between the two ends of the suture thread forming a 'V' (Fig 5.53)
2. Loop the thread attached to the needle around the needle holder 3 times in a clock-wise fashion (Fig 5.54). Keep hold of this long end of the suture
3. Grasp the very tip of the short end of the suture (from the original insertion site) with the needle holder. Pull the two ends of sutures in opposite directions at right angles to the wound forming the first knot (Fig 5.55)
4. Form a 'V' shape with the two ends of the suture (Fig 5.56) Then place the needle holder in between the two ends
5. Loop the thread attached to the needle around the needle holder two times in an anti-clockwise fashion. (Fig 5.57) Grasp the very tip of the short end of the suture with the needle holder. Pull the two ends of sutures in opposite directions at right angles to the wound. This is the second knot
6. Follow steps 1 – 3 above to lay down the third knot
7. Reposition your knots so that they are not lying over the line of the wound (Fig 5.58)
8. Cut the ends of the suture, leaving approximately 5mm each end (Fig 5.59). Ensure the suture needle is immediately disposed in a sharps bin
9. Repeat steps 1 – 8 above 5-10mm on both sides along from your first suture (Fig 5.60)
10. Ensure that all the wound edges are successfully brought together

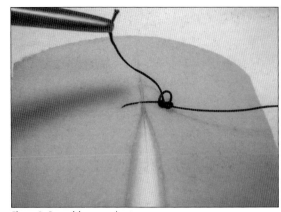
Fig 5.58: Reposition your knot

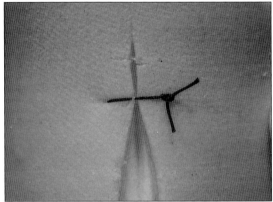
Fig 5.59: An uninterrupted suture

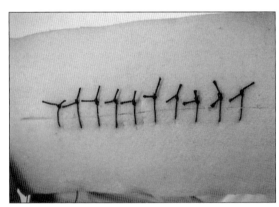
Fig 5.60: A series of uninterrupted sutures

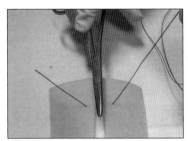
Fig 5.53: The first "V"

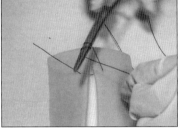
Fig 5.54: Looping the suture

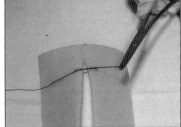
Fig 5.55: The first knot

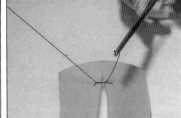
Fig 5.56: The second "V"

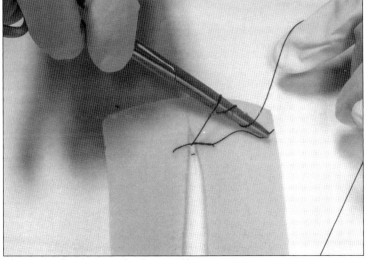
Fig 5.57: Looping the suture for the second knot

'Use the forceps to grip the needle with the needle holder; never handle the needle with your fingers'

'Each successive knot should be laid down in opposite directions; as this pattern prevents the suture from unravelling'

MEDICINE AND SURGERY

Documenting the Procedure

Document under the following headings:
- Details of site of laceration and wound assessment
- Any referrals made
- Amount of LA used
- Wound suturing performed on patient
- Complications
- Estimated blood loss
- Any subsequent tests ordered
- Details of follow up and wound after care

Wound After Care

- Apply a dressing over the wound if required
- Always administer a tetanus booster if the patient has not had one in the past 10 years or if the wound is contaminated
- Advise the patient to keep the wound dry whilst showering/washing
- Educate the patient on signs of wound infection (e.g. redness, soreness, discharge) and advise them to seek medical help if this occurs

Different Aspects of Sutures

Absorbable	Non-Absorbable	Monofilament	Polyfilament
• Are naturally dissolved by the body and hence do not need to be removed • Are more likely to leave a pronounced scar when used on skin • May be useful in children who are expected to be distressed during suture removal	• Are less tissue reactive and therefore leave less scarring • Typically used for skin suturing and removed in a health care setting during wound check • May be useful in children who are expected to be distressed during suture removal	• Recommended for skin closures • Decreased risk of infection compared to polyfilament	• Made of many strands of thread twisted together • Are easier to tie than monofilament • The micro-spaces in between the threads allow for easier bacterial colonisation compared to monofilament

Mark Scheme for Examiner

Introduction and General Advice

Introduces self (clean hands)

Identifies patient (3 points of ID)

Explains procedure, identifies concerns, checks allergies, and obtains consent

Inspects and assesses wound site

Discusses referral to specialist surgeons if appropriate

Preparation

Obtains equipment and checks expiry dates

Washes hands, dons sterile gloves

Injects LA using the 'withdraw and infiltrate' method

Cleans wound site with sterile water and iodine solution

Suturing

Inserts needle perpendicular to skin at correct distance ☐ ☐ ☐ ☐ ☐

Withdraws needle with forceps from the centre of the wound ☐ ☐ ☐ ☐ ☐

Re-enters wound parallel to original insertion ☐ ☐ ☐ ☐ ☐

Pulls suture thread taut with forceps ☐ ☐ ☐ ☐ ☐

Ties three knots for each suture and repositions knot ☐ ☐ ☐ ☐ ☐

Ensures wound edges are successfully brought together ☐ ☐ ☐ ☐ ☐

Finishing

Places dressing over wound ☐ ☐ ☐ ☐ ☐

Disposes of equipment ☐ ☐ ☐ ☐ ☐

Removes gloves and wash hands ☐ ☐ ☐ ☐ ☐

Documents procedure in patient notes ☐ ☐ ☐ ☐ ☐

General Points

Talks throughout the procedure to the patient ☐ ☐ ☐ ☐ ☐

Disposes of all sharps immediately ☐ ☐ ☐ ☐ ☐

Avoids patient contamination (i.e. NTT) ☐ ☐ ☐ ☐ ☐

Questions and Answers for Candidate

Name some alternatives to suturing

- Steri-strips
- Staples
- Tissue adhesives (glue)

When are non-absorbable sutures removed?

- Sutures will normally be removed in 7-14 days (4-5 days in the case of the face); this can usually be done with the agreement of their GP or district nurse

When is a mattress suture indicated?

- When the skin edges are difficult to evert. They provide good dermis-to-dermis contact and can be used in conjunction with simple interrupted sutures
- When a wound is not holding together, for example if the wound edges are under tension

Additional Questions to Consider

1. When would you refer to a specialist for suturing a wound?
2. When would you give a patient with a wound a tetanus booster?
3. How might you get a child to remain still when suturing a wound?

Station 13: SURGICAL GOWNING AND GLOVING

You have been asked to assist in surgery. Scrub up using an aseptic technique.

Objectives

- Scrub up aseptically
- Maintain a sterile field

General Advice

- Always ask if you are unsure about touching objects in the operating theatre; this will help maintain sterility
- It is important not to touch sterile gowns or gloves when opening their packets as this results in contamination
- The accepted clothing underneath a surgical gown are surgical scrubs with comfortable theatre shoes and these should not be worn outside of the hospital
- Nails should be short and without nail polish
- Rings, watches, jewellery, wallets and mobile phones should be locked away out of the operating theatre

Equipment Checklist

(Fig 5.61)

a) Surgical cap
b) Face mask ± eye shield
c) Theatre shoes/boots
d) Sink with elbow tap handles and elbow activated antiseptic wash
e) Sterile paper towels
f) Hand scrubber packet (including brush and sponge)
g) Gowning trolley
h) Correctly sized sterile gown
i) Correctly sized sterile gloves
j) An assistant

Scrubbing up Procedures

Non-Sterile Procedures

1. Wear a surgical cap before entering the surgical scrubbing room. This should be tied so that any falling hair is trapped in the cap. Put on theatre shoes

2. Wash hands at the sink inside the scrubbing room and dry with paper towels nearby

3. Tie on a face mask ± eye shield (depending on the type of surgery) ensuring that it covers both mouth and nose (Fig 5.62)

4. Find the gowning trolley and obtain the sterile gown, don't collect the gloves yet

5. Open the packet containing the surgical gown in an aseptic fashion and drop it facing upwards on the gowning trolley gently

6. Opening the packet should reveal a surgical gown below sterile paper towels. Obtain hand scrubber packet

7. Open a packet of sterile gloves (of the appropriate size), placing them so that you still have access to the sterile paper towels

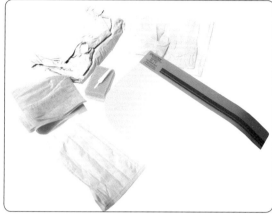
Fig 5.61: Open all equipment you require before starting to scrub

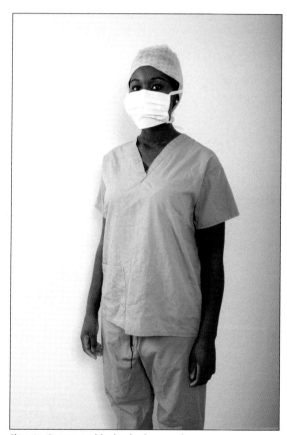
Fig 5.62: Correct positioning for face mask

'It helps to pinch the nose bridge of the face mask to allow a more comfortable fit. Ensuring that the face mask fits well is of critical importance as it is not sterile and therefore cannot be adjusted by you after starting to scrub up'

First Wash Technique

1. Open the tap to get the water flowing at a comfortable temperature and rate which avoids splashing. **You must not touch the taps with your hands after this step**

2. Wet hands up to elbows, ensuring that water is flowing from the fingers down to the elbows throughout the procedure (Fig 5.63)

3. Open the hand scrubber packet and use the pick inside to remove any dirt/debris from under the nails then discard the pick into a nearby bin

4. Press the lever of the antiseptic bottle with the elbow of one arm whilst positioning the hand of the other arm under the bottle to receive the solution onto the sponge part of the scrubber

5. Use the sponge to clean the fingernails, palms, back of hands, wrists, forearms thoroughly and work downwards to the elbows (Fig 5.64)

6. Discard the sponge into a nearby bin and then wash the hands up to elbows

Second Wash Technique

1. Press the lever of the antiseptic bottle with the elbow of one arm whilst positioning the hand of the other arm under the bottle to receive the solution onto the other hand

2. Wash hands according to the WHO guidelines (see station 8.1)

3. Rotationally rub the wrist, working down to the elbows with one hand and then vice versa

4. Wash the hands up to elbows in a 'swinging motion'

Third Wash Technique

1. Perform exactly the same wash for both arms but stop two-thirds down the forearm, not reaching the elbows

2. Place your arms bent at the elbow in front of you and allow the water to drip off your elbows (Fig 5.65)

3. Close the tap with your elbow, taking care to minimizing contact as much as possible

4. Return to the gowning trolley and use one paper towel per arm, drying from fingertips to elbows in a dabbing motion. **Do not go back and dry in the opposite direction.** Discard the paper towel once used and repeat for the other arm (Fig 5.66 and 5.67)

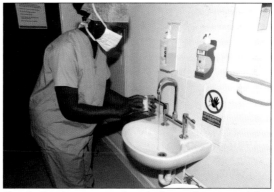

Fig 5.64: Use the sponge to clean the fingernails more carefully

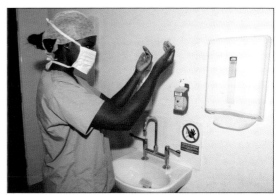

Fig 5.65: Remember that you are now sterile and should avoid any contamination

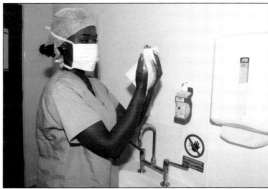

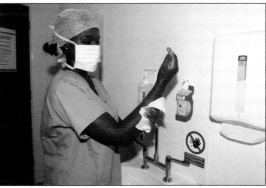

Fig 5.66 and 5.67: Always start drying from the hands

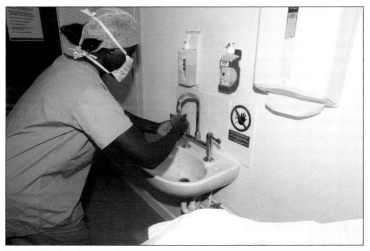

Fig 5.63: Wet hands up to elbows

Scrubbing Up

1. Arrange your hands so your fingers are close together and thumbs are pointing upwards. Place each hand in the arm holes of the gown (Fig 5.68)

2. Lift the gown

3. Holding the gown gently but firmly, step back from the trolley ensuring there is no equipment nearby

4. Extend your elbows from your body and move your arms apart. The gown should open itself and you will be able to slip your hands and arms in the gown (Fig 5.69)

5. Do not let your hands go beyond the cuff

6. Ask an assistant to fasten your neck collar and ties at the back

> 'Ensure that your hands stay inside the gown; do not use them to drape the gown over. Your bare hands should not go beyond the gown cuffs at any point or touch the outside of the glove'

Donning Gloves using the 'Closed Glove Technique'

1. Gripping through the gown cuffs, place the glove packet upside down

2. Unfold the packet via gripping its edges. The right glove should now be on the left and the left glove on the right

3. Grasp the folded cuff of the right glove with the right hand (Fig 5.70)

4. Pick the right glove up and rest it on your right hand. The fingers of the glove should be pointing towards your body, the palm should be facing outwards and the thumb should not be visible as it is resting on your hand (Fig 5.71)

5. Whilst keeping your grip on the folded cuff with your right hand, use your left hand (through the gown's cuff) to grab the other folded cuff, which is facing you (Fig 5.72)

6. Bring the cuff of the glove facing you over the fingers of your right hand and slide your right hand into the glove (Fig 5.73)

7. Unroll the rest of the glove to allow it to fit more securely and comfortably on your right hand. Then straighten the gown so the cuffs cover a little more than your wrist (Fig 5.74)

8. Follow steps above for the left hand

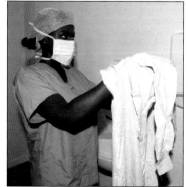

Fig 5.68: Remember that the gown is also sterile and should not touch any surface

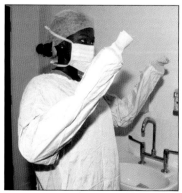

Fig 5.69: Straighten your arms

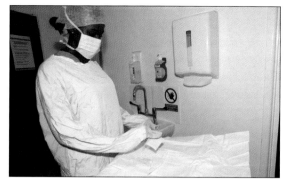

Fig 5.70: Putting on sterile gloves, correct preparation

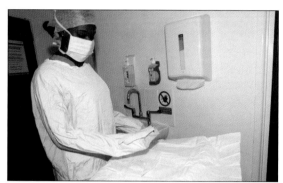

Fig 5.71: Flip the glove so it is facing you

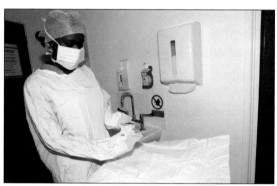

Fig 5.72: Grip the glove

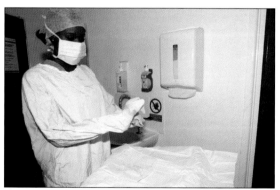

Fig 5.73: Slide your hand in the glove

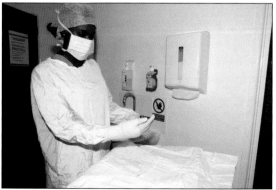

Fig 5.74: Now position the glove

Securing the Gown

1. Find the piece of card with two ties attached. This is called the 'dance card' (Fig 5.75)
2. Hold onto the short tie with your left hand and remove it from the gown. Do not let go of the short tie
3. Give the dance card with the right tie attached to the assistant, ensuring that there is no hand contact (Fig 5.76)
4. Let go of the dance card and turn around 360° anti-clockwise (Fig 5.77)
5. Grip the tie and pull away from the card held by the assistant
6. Tie a simple reef knot with the ties in your left and right hand (Fig 5.78)
7. Keep your hands near your chest to ensure you remain sterile (Fig 5.79)

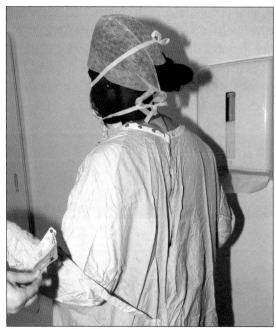

Fig 5.77: Turn fully whilst your assistant holds the 'dance card'

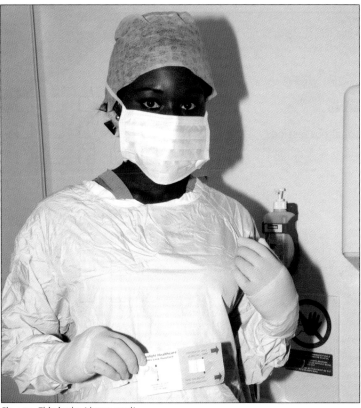

Fig 5.75: This is the 'dance card'

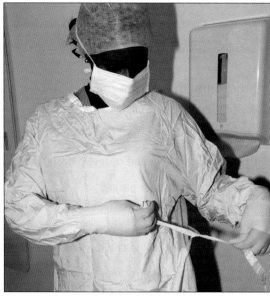

Fig 5.78: Secure your gown in place by forming a knot

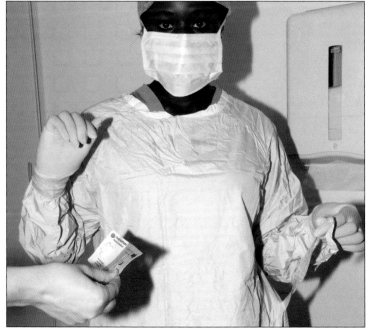

Fig 5.76: Hand the 'dance card' to your assistant

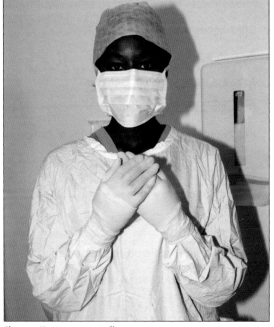

Fig 5.79: You are now sterile

Mrs Manpreet is a 35-year-old female who presents to your clinic with abdominal pain and vomiting. She has been going to the toilet more often than normal, and when she does pass urine, it stings. She is also concerned that her urine is foul-smelling. Please ask her to provide a mid-stream urine sample, perform a urinalysis on it and discuss the results with her.

Objectives

- Explaining mid-stream urine samples
- Performing urinalysis
- Interpret urinalysis findings

Equipment Checklist

(remember to check expiry dates on all equipment) (Fig 6.1)

a) Non-sterile gloves
b) Urine reagent strip
c) Sterile urine pot
d) Paper towel

General Advice

- Obtain consent
- Where possible, it is important to obtain a fresh urine sample for analysis
- Ensure that when you interpret the urinalysis findings, you take into consideration the patient's signs and symptoms
- If you are going to throw the urine sample away after analysis, ensure this is down a sluice and not a domestic sink

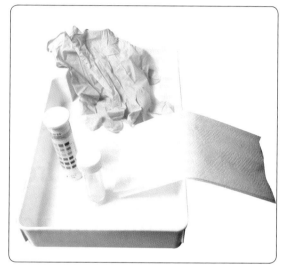

Fig 6.1: Equipment required to perform urinalysis

Obtaining a Mid-Stream Urine Sample

1. Give the patient a sterile midstream urine pot – this usually contains boric acid
2. Ask them to clean their external genitalia with water and tissue
3. Ask them to pass a small amount of urine into the toilet
4. Then, without stopping the flow of urine, catch some into the pot to fill to the line
5. Advise the patient that he/she can empty his/her bladder into the toilet
6. Immediately place the cap onto the urine pot

Performing a Urine Dipstick

1. Give the patient a sterile universal pot and ask them to provide a urine sample
2. Wash your hands
3. Put on gloves
4. Inspect the urine sample – does it look cloudy, dark yellow, red or have any sediment?
5. Remove the cap of the urine container – note any smell
6. Check the expiry date of the dipstick on the container and remove one dipstick
7. Place the dipstick in the urine for 2-3 seconds, ensuring that all the reagents on the dipstick are immersed in the urine (Fig 6.2)

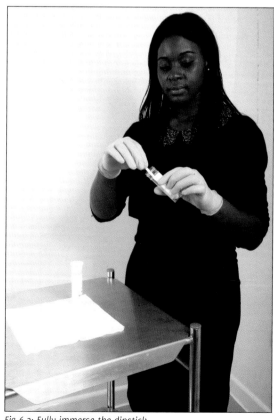

Fig 6.2: Fully immerse the dipstick

8. Remove the dipstick

9. Place the dipstick horizontally onto a flat surface/paper towel to ensure that the chemicals do not mix (Fig 6.3)

10. Leave the dipstick to dry for the specified time (found on the reagent strip container)

11. Look at each reagent on the dipstick in turn. With each reagent, look at the corresponding colour on the tub (the tub will have a colour code on its side so that you can interpret the results) and identify if the value is normal or high (Fig 6.4)

12. Document the findings in the patient notes and report back to the patient

Finishing

1. Label the pot and accompanying laboratory form with patient details and send to the lab

2. Remove gloves and wash hands

3. Discuss your findings with the patient

Interpretation

All of the results need to be interpreted in the context of the patient. A raised glucose on urinalysis does not necessarily mean that the patient has diabetes. For example, glycosuria can be normal in the context of pregnancy

Appearance	Inference
• Red	Can indicate haematuria
• Cloudy	Can indicate infection
• Faeculent	Colovesical fistula or contaminated sample
Smell	
• Foul	Infection
• Sweet	Diabetic ketoacidosis (DKA)
• Faeculent	Colovesical fistula or contaminated sample
Blood	
• Positive	Haematuria or haemoglobinuria
• False positive	Menstrual blood
Ketones	
• Raised	DKA, starvation
Nitrites and Leucocytes	
• Both positive	Suggests bacterial infection
• Nitrites positive	Suggests bacterial infection
• Leucocytes positive	Suggests inflammation and possible infection

Continues overleaf...

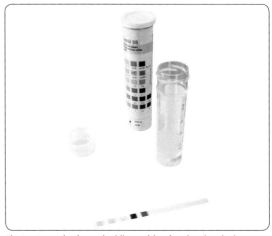

Fig 6.3: Leave horizontal whilst waiting for the chemicals to react

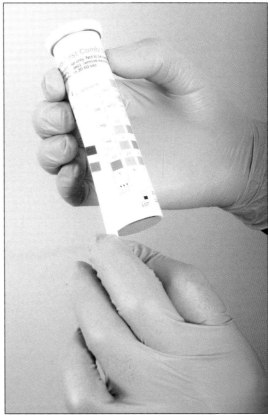

Fig 6.4: Interpret the results using the chart on the dip stick bottle

If the patient is unable to pass urine and requires catheterisation, a sample may be obtained when the catheter is inserted

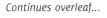

UROLOGY

Protein

Raised	Renovascular, glomerular or tubulo-interstitial renal disease Pre-eclampsia and hypertension Benign due to exercise or postural Nephrotic syndrome

Glucose

Raised	Diabetes, pregnancy and some patients on steroids

Specific Gravity

High value	Dehydration, heart failure, liver failure and syndrome of inappropriate ADH (SiADH)
Low value	Diabetes insipidus and increased fluid intake

pH

Alkaline	Can indicate UTI with urea splitting organisms (e.g. Proteus)
Acidic	Can indicate urinary stones made of uric acid and cystine

'Don't throw away a urine sample after the dipstick is done: wait until a decision is made as to whether it needs to be sent for further investigation'

Present Your Findings

Mrs Manpreet is a 35-year-old female who presented with symptoms of a urinary tract infection. Urinalysis demonstrated nitrites+++ leucocytes++ blood+ therefore, I have started her on a course of trimethoprim and sent her urine sample away for MC&S

Further Urine Investigations

- A pregnancy test is important in all fertile women presenting with abdominal pain
- If there is evidence of a urinary tract infection (leukocytes, nitrites, blood, protein) send the urine sample for MC&S
- If there is a concern about myeloma (bone pain, anaemia, renal failure, elevated calcium, proteinuria), send the urine for protein electrophoresis
- Urine microscopy can reveal red-cell casts. These occur in the context of glomerulonephritis. In this setting, you need to inform the lab that you are specifically looking for pathological casts on microscopy and the sample will be analysed as soon as practical after being produced, ideally whilst still warm
- Urine can be tested for microalbuminuria in patients that have diabetes mellitus (newer dipsticks can measure this). This is a screening test for nephropathy
- Protein to creatinine ratios (or urinary PCRs) are useful in quantifying the extent of a patient's proteinuria. A patient has nephrotic range proteinuria when they are passing more than 3 g per 24 hours

Mark Scheme for Examiner

Introduction and General Advice

Introduces self (clean hands)	☐	☐	☐	☐	☐
Identifies patient (3 points of ID)	☐	☐	☐	☐	☐
Explains procedure, identifies concerns and obtains consent	☐	☐	☐	☐	☐

Obtaining Mid-Stream Urine Sample

Provides patient with sterile specimen pot	☐	☐	☐	☐	☐
Asks for a mid-stream urine sample	☐	☐	☐	☐	☐
Explains how to collect a mid-stream urine sample	☐	☐	☐	☐	☐

Urine Dipstick

Washes hands, dons non-sterile gloves	⌐	⌐	⌐	⌐	⌐
Checks expiry date of reagent sticks	⌐	⌐	⌐	⌐	⌐
Inspects sample	⌐	⌐	⌐	⌐	⌐
Removes cap and notes odour	⌐	⌐	⌐	⌐	⌐
Removes a single dipstick from container	⌐	⌐	⌐	⌐	⌐
Dips the urine for 2-3 seconds	⌐	⌐	⌐	⌐	⌐
Places dipstick on flat surface and leave for specified time	⌐	⌐	⌐	⌐	⌐
Uses the colour chart of dipstick container to analyse results	⌐	⌐	⌐	⌐	⌐

Finishing

If indicated, sends sample away, otherwise disposes of sample	⌐	⌐	⌐	⌐	⌐
Removes gloves and washes hands	⌐	⌐	⌐	⌐	⌐
Disposes of equipment and cleans work surface	⌐	⌐	⌐	⌐	⌐

Interpretation

Comments on: blood; ketones; nitrites; leucocytes; protein; glucose; specific gravity and pH	⌐	⌐	⌐	⌐	⌐
Discusses the dipstick findings in relation to the patient's symptoms	⌐	⌐	⌐	⌐	⌐
Documents findings and management plan in patient notes	⌐	⌐	⌐	⌐	⌐

Questions and Answers for Candidate

When might you get a false-positive glucose test on a urine dip?

- The presence of other substances in the urine can interfere with the test strips and give a false positive
- Examples include aspirin, penicillin, isoniazid, vitamin C and cephalosporins

What does the presence of red cell casts on light microscopy suggest?

- Glomerulonephritis

Give 8 causes of haematuria

- Kidney: malignancy; calculi; trauma; glomerulonephritis; pyelonephritis; interstitial nephritis; infarction; polycystic kidney disease
- Ureter: malignancy; calculi; trauma
- Bladder: malignancy; calculi; trauma; infection
- Urethra and prostate: malignancy; stone; trauma; benign prostatic hypertrophy (BPH)
- General: anticoagulants, e.g. warfarin; exercise; paroxysmal nocturnal haematuria
- Not true haematuria: May purely be vaginal bleeding/ menstruation. May not be blood at all (beetroot can give similar appearance, as can certain drugs, e.g. rifampicin)

What methods are available for collecting urine samples in a baby?

- Clean-catch urine: Waiting for urination with a sterile pot after the nappy has been removed and the surrounding area has been cleaned (parents should be told to ask for a new sterile pot if it gets contaminated)
- Supra-pubic aspiration (ultrasound guided)
- Catheter sample

Additional Questions to Consider

1. What are urinary Bence Jones proteins?
2. Name some causes of proteinuria
3. What bacteria are commonly associated with staghorn calculi?
4. Is there a difference in the length of antibiotic course for a simple UTI in men compared to women?
5. How would pyelonephritis present and how would you treat it?

UROLOGY

Mr Gear has not urinated following an elective operation he had last night and is becoming distressed by abdominal pain. An examination reveals a soft non-tender suprapubic mass which, when palpated deeply, makes Mr Gear feel like he wishes to pass urine. You diagnose acute urinary retention and feel that he requires a urethral catheter. Having already obtained his consent, demonstrate this procedure on the mannequin provided.

Objectives

- Learn how to perform male catheterisation

General Advice

- Confirm that the patient understands what is going to happen and is happy to continue
- Obtain valid consent
- Always ask for a chaperone

Catheter Selection

Size: Use the smallest catheter you can. Normally 14 Ch is used in males and 12 Ch in females
Length: A male catheter is approximately 40 cm; a female catheter is approximately 25 cm
Material: Silicone or hydrogel (lasts up to 3 months) or coated latex (lasts up to 4 weeks). Remember to ask about allergies; a patient with latex allergies should have an all silicone catheter and you should use non-latex gloves

> 'Make sure you carefully select the right catheter for your patient, paying particular attention to the length. You must never use a female catheter in a male patient'

Equipment Checklist

(remember to check expiry dates on all equipment) (Fig 6.5)

a) Procedure trolley
b) Sharps bin
c) Disposable bag (for rubbish)
d) Catheterisation pack (including disposable dish, plastic pots, cotton swabs and sterile drape)
e) 2 × sterile water/0.9% saline sachets, according to Trust policy
f) 2 x pairs sterile gloves
g) LA gel or lubricant, according to Trust policy
h) 21-gauge needle
i) 10 mL syringe
j) Sterile water vial (often pre-drawn up with the catheter)
k) Large incontinence pad
l) Single use disposable apron
m) Male catheter
n) Catheter bag (leg bag if appropriate for the patient)
o) Sterile universal container (if collecting urine sample)

Causes of Urinary Retention

Bladder
- Detrusor problems
- Bladder tumours
- Neurogenic bladder (e.g. spinal injuries, Parkinson's syndrome or Multiple Sclerosis)
- Damage to the bladder and bladder neck

Prostatic
- Benign prostatic hypertrophy
- Prostatic cancer
- Prostatitis

Penile
- Congenital urethral valves
- Phimosis
- Obstruction (e.g. tumour, stone or a stricture)

Other
- Pelvic malignancy
- Constipation
- Metastases
- Post-operatively
- Drugs (e.g. anticholinergics or psychoactive drugs)

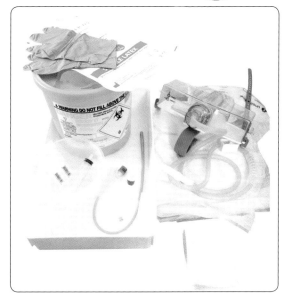

Fig 6.5: Ensure you prepare your equipment

Explaining Catheterisation to the Patient

1. A urinary catheter is a tube that is placed into the bladder through the hole in the end of your penis, called the urethra, and attached to a bag that collects the urine
2. You will need to be exposed from your belly button to your knees and lie with your legs slightly apart
3. Initially, the genitalia will be cleaned and then some anaesthetic gel will be inserted into the urethral meatus to make the procedure more comfortable
4. The catheter will then be inserted and held in place using a balloon
5. It is really important that if you feel any pain that you tell a nurse or doctor immediately

Performing Catheterisation

Prepare Procedure Trolley

1. Clean your hands
2. Clean the trolley according to local policy
3. Place a sharps bin on the bottom of your trolley
4. Open a disposable rubbish bag and attach it to the side of the trolley
5. Gather your equipment and check the expiry dates
6. Open the catheterisation pack using a sterile NTT on the centre of trolley
7. Then open the packaging and drop the lubricant, sachets, gloves and catheter onto the aseptic field
8. Open the packaging of the catheter bag
9. If not pre-prepared, draw up sterile water using a 21-gauge needle and a 10 mL syringe. After use, place the needle in the sharps bin

Prepare the Patient

1. Expose and position the patient supine but keep them covered with a blanket or towel until just before the procedure, ensuring patient dignity
2. Put the incontinence pad under the patient
3. Wash your hands thoroughly, put on a single use disposable apron and put on sterile gloves
4. Place a sterile drape with central hole over the penis (leaving the penis exposed)

Asepsis and Anaesthesia

1. Ask assistant to empty both sterile water sachets into plastic pot
2. Soak the cotton swabs in water
3. Hold the penis with the non-dominant hand and retract the prepuce/foreskin. This hand is contaminated and should now not touch the aseptic trolley
4. With the right hand, clean the penis in circles beginning at the urethra and moving progressively outwards. Repeat this at least 3 times
5. Dispose of the swabs in disposable rubbish bag
6. Holding the penis in the non-dominant hand, apply some upwards traction and insert the tip of the lubricant syringe into the urethral meatus (Fig 6.6)
7. Administer the entire lubricant syringe, allowing some to coat the glans
8. Leave the lubricant for five minutes to take effect
9. Remove gloves, wash hands and put on second pair of sterile gloves

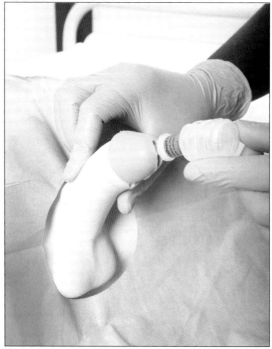

Fig 6.6: Use anaesthetic gel prior to catheter insertion

Inserting the Catheter

1. Place the disposable dish between the patient's legs so that once the catheter is in, urine does not spill onto the bed sheets
2. Hold the catheter between your thumb and forefinger in your dominant hand
3. Hold the base of the penis with the non-dominant hand. Apply gentle upward traction to the penis, while inserting the catheter with the other hand into the urethral meatus
4. Insert the catheter using a NTT by touching only the packaging, i.e. insert directly from sterilised packaging (without taking the catheter completely out of the packaging) (Fig 6.7)

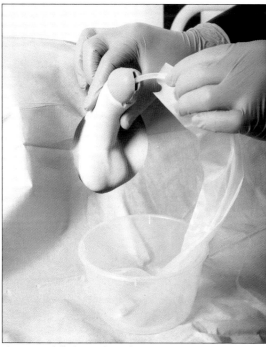

Fig 6.7: Carefully insert the catheter

UROLOGY

5. Use steady gentle pressure and never force a catheter
6. Advance the catheter until urine is seen to flow into the container
7. Then, once urine is seen to be draining, advance the catheter by another 2.5cm
8. If no urine is seen draining, advance the catheter to the fork at the end
9. Attach the sterile water syringe to the balloon port of the catheter and insert 10 mL slowly. STOP if there is pain or high resistance (Fig 6.8)
10. Attach the catheter to the catheter bag by removing the cap from the tubing and plugging the plastic tube end into the catheter (Fig 6.9)
11. Replace the prepuce
12. If there is a leg-bag, attach it to the leg. Larger collection bags may be attached to the side of the patient's bed
13. Clean the patient, remove the incontinence pad and ensure dignity by rearranging bed-clothes
14. Dispose of waste
15. Clean the trolley according to local policy
16. Remove gloves and decontaminate hands
17. Tell the patient to report any pain or other concerns to the nursing staff
18. Document insertion of catheter

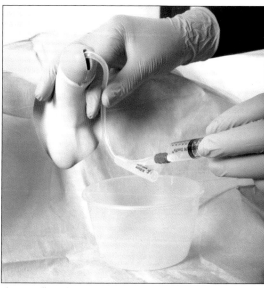

Fig 6.8: Inflate the balloon using sterile water into the side-port

Documenting the Procedure

You need to document the procedure in the medical notes (often a sticker from catheter pack is provided for this purpose). Document the procedure writing the following points:

- Consent obtained and chaperone present
- Date and time of insertion
- Reason for insertion
- Size, length and material of catheter
- Ease with which catheter passed
- Colour of urine drained
- Volume of sterile water inserted into balloon
- Residual volume of urine (5-10 minutes after insertion)
- Sign and print your name under your entry

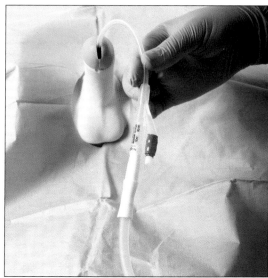

Fig 6.9: Attach the drainage bag

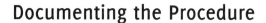

Mark Scheme for Examiner

Introduction and General Advice

Introduces self (clean hands)

Identifies patient (3 points of ID)

Ensures that consent has been obtained

Explains procedure and identify concerns

Asks for a chaperone

Positions and exposes the patient

Chooses the correct size, material and type of catheter

Procedure Preparation

Cleans hands ☐ ☐ ☐ ☐ ☐

Obtains equipment and checks expiry dates ☐ ☐ ☐ ☐ ☐

Cleans the trolley ☐ ☐ ☐ ☐ ☐

Prepares trolley and equipment ☐ ☐ ☐ ☐ ☐

If not provided, draws up sterile water into a syringe using a green needle ☐ ☐ ☐ ☐ ☐

Procedure

Washes hands, dons sterile gloves and apron ☐ ☐ ☐ ☐ ☐

Places sterile drape leaving the central hole for the penis ☐ ☐ ☐ ☐ ☐

Asks assistant to put sterile water into the plastic pot ☐ ☐ ☐ ☐ ☐

Cleans the genitalia including the urethral opening ☐ ☐ ☐ ☐ ☐

Administers the lubricant correctly ☐ ☐ ☐ ☐ ☐

Removes gloves, washes hands and puts on second pair of sterile gloves ☐ ☐ ☐ ☐ ☐

Places disposable dish between the legs to catch the urine ☐ ☐ ☐ ☐ ☐

Holds the penis in the non-dominant hand and applies upward traction ☐ ☐ ☐ ☐ ☐

Inserts the catheter slowly using a NTT until urine passes into the dish
or pain/resistance is experienced ☐ ☐ ☐ ☐ ☐

Inflates the balloon with 10 mL sterile water (asks if this is painful and stops if it is) ☐ ☐ ☐ ☐ ☐

Connects catheter to catheter bag ☐ ☐ ☐ ☐ ☐

Replaces the prepuce ☐ ☐ ☐ ☐ ☐

Washes hands ☐ ☐ ☐ ☐ ☐

Informs patient to inform someone if any pain occurs ☐ ☐ ☐ ☐ ☐

Documents the procedure in the notes ☐ ☐ ☐ ☐ ☐

General Points

Continuous communication with the patient throughout the procedure ☐ ☐ ☐ ☐ ☐

Aseptic technique throughout ☐ ☐ ☐ ☐ ☐

Disposes of sharps and clinical waste appropriately ☐ ☐ ☐ ☐ ☐

UROLOGY

UROLOGY
UROLOGY

7 PAEDIATRICS

PAEDIATRICS

Station 1: PEAK FLOW

Mrs Patel has come to your clinic with her 14-year-old son, Sandeep. He has recently been diagnosed with asthma, and has been advised to keep a peak flow diary. Please teach him how to perform a peak flow.

Objectives

- Learn how to perform peak flow
- Explain peak flow monitoring

General Advice

- Ensure that you have introduced yourself, identified the patient and washed your hands
- Ensure that your patient has given verbal consent for the procedure and is happy for family/friends present to remain
- Always make sure there are spare mouth pieces available for the next patient
- When the patient is given a peak flow monitor they will have their own mouthpiece that they can reuse and wash

Explaining the Procedure to the Patient

- People who have been diagnosed with asthma have difficulties with breathing
- A peak flow monitor can demonstrate how well controlled asthma is over a particular period of time by showing how much air can be exhaled out of the lungs quickly
- The technique of how to use the peak flow monitor will be demonstrated before you are asked to use it

Equipment

a) Peak flow monitor
b) Disposable mouth piece

How to Perform Peak Flow

After demonstrating peak flow to the patient, ask them to perform the procedure without instruction to check understanding and technique. Language used may need to be adjusted depending on the child's level of understanding

1. Ask the patient to stand up or sit up straight
2. Ensure that the dial on the peak flow monitor is at ZERO (Fig 7.1)
3. Make sure that the patient knows not to let their fingers touch the scale or markers during use (Fig 7.2)
4. Ask the patient to fit the mouthpiece onto the monitor, making sure there is a tight seal around the mouthpiece
5. Ask the patient to inhale deeply
6. Ask the patient to place his lips firmly around the mouthpiece
7. Advise the patient to lift his chin and straighten their back to open their airways fully
8. Advise the patient to blow out as hard and as fast as he can. You can use phrases such as 'like you are blowing out the candles on a cake' (Fig 7.3)

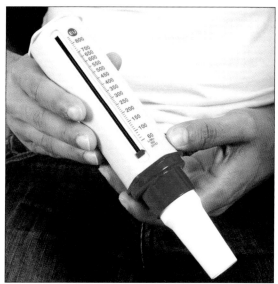
Fig 7.1: Prepare the peak flow monitor before use

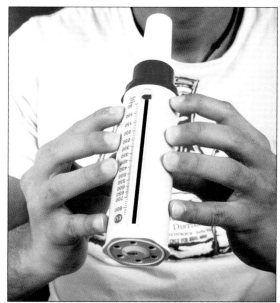
Fig 7.2: Hold the peak flow meter correctly

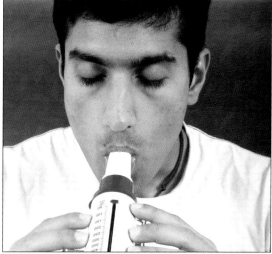
Fig 7.3: Ask the patient to blow out as hard and as fast as he can

9. Check the dial, record the reading (Fig 7.4)
10. Move the dial back to zero
11. Allow the patient a period of rest and then repeat the procedure. It should be performed 3 times and the highest value is the one taken as the peak flow reading at that time
12. Compare the reading to a standard chart
13. Record the results in a peak flow diary and explain to the patient how to use it

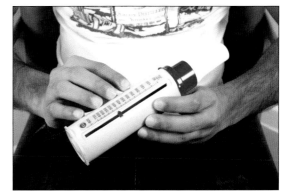

Fig 7.4: Check the reading for the patient

You express the PEFR as % of the patient's best (if known) or predicted best according to their sex and height
For asthma, the PEFR is useful to assess the patient's condition and helps determine how you are going to treat them:
- >75% = mild/moderate state
- <50% = severe state
- <33% = life threatening state

Mark Scheme for Examiner

Introduction and General Advice

Introduces self (clean hands)

Identifies patient (3 points of ID)

Ensures that consent has been obtained

Checks identity of others in the room and confirms that the patient is happy for them to stay

Explains the procedure and identify concerns

Explaining Peak Flow

Describes the technique of using the peak flow monitor

Mentions it should be done three times

Watches the patient do it without instruction

Discusses the use of a peak flow diary

Finishing the Consultation

Elicits patient concerns and questions

Arranges a follow up appointment if necessary or offers contact details

Thanks the patient and closes the consultation

General Points

Checks patient understanding throughout the consultation, avoiding medical jargon, and offers information leaflets

Maintains good eye contact; remains polite and engaged with the patient

PAEDIATRICS

Questions and Answers for Candidate

What factors affect the peak flow result?

- Quality of peak flow technique
- Degree of lung disease
- Height, age and gender

Why is a peak flow diary useful?

- To establish if there is diurnal variation in peak flow associated with asthma
- To establish if there are any environmental triggers associated with asthma

What are the typical changes in lung spirometry in asthma?

- If there is an obstructive defect
- o The FEV_1 is reduced
- o The FEV_1/FVC is reduced
- o >15% improvement in FEV_1 following a B_2 agonist or steroid trial, demonstrating reversibility of airway constriction

Additional Questions to Consider

1. What age group can peak flow be used for?
2. What is the British Thoracic Society's step-wise approach to management in asthma and when do you move up or down a step?
3. What are the differences between a severe and life-threatening asthma attack?
4. What would be your initial management in an acute asthma attack?

Station 2: INHALER TECHNIQUE

Mrs Page has come to your clinic with her 7-year-old son, Toby. He has recently been diagnosed with asthma and has been given inhalers. Please teach him how to use an inhaler and a spacer.

Objectives

- Learn inhaler technique
- Learn how to use a spacer device

Explaining the Inhalers to the Patient

- People who have been diagnosed with asthma use inhalers to help with their breathing. Some inhalers are used every day and some are just used when the patient gets wheezy or thinks they will get wheezy
- The different colours of the inhalers show that they do different things: (Fig 7.5)
  - o The blue inhaler is a reliever and should be used when the patient is wheezy as he will feel an immediate improvement in his breathing. If he uses this more than three times a week, he needs to see his GP
  - o The brown/orange inhaler is a preventer and should be used regularly. He will not notice a difference quickly with this inhaler, but it helps in the long term
  - o Other colours may mean that the inhaler contains two different types of medication e.g. a purple inhaler

Inhaler Technique

After demonstrating inhaler technique to the patient, ask him to perform the procedure without instruction to check understanding and technique. Language used may need to be adjusted dependent on the child's level of understanding

1. Check the expiry date of the inhaler
2. Ask the patient to stand up or sit up straight and lift his chin
3. Shake the inhaler well
4. Take the cap off the inhaler (Fig 7.6)
5. Ask the patient to exhale completely
6. Ask the patient to place his lips firmly around the mouthpiece (Fig 7.7)
7. Ask the patient to press the canister as he starts to inhale slowly. Remove inhaler from mouth
8. Ask the patient to hold his breath for ten seconds and then breath out slowly
9. If more than one puff is required, wait ten seconds before repeating the process

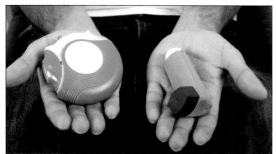

Fig 7.5: Inhalers come in all shapes and sizes

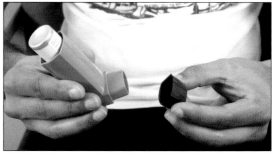

Fig 7.6: Prepare the inhaler for use

- Inhalers last for about 200 puffs
- The inhalers have a use-by-date printed on the side; if this expires, a new inhaler is needed
- If the child is using their inhaler more than 3 times a week he needs to see his GP to assess his treatment options
- It is important that you inform patients that they must rinse their mouth out after using steroid inhalers to reduce the risk of oral candida

'Encourage patients to carry a blue reliever inhaler with them as well as having one at home as it is hard to predict when they become symptomatic'

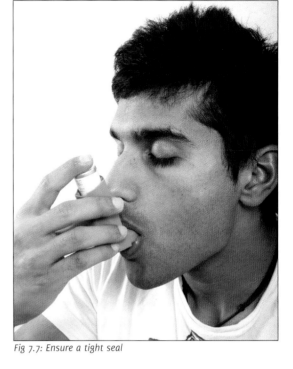
Fig 7.7: Ensure a tight seal

Using a Spacer

It is important to explain the advantages of using a spacer; i.e. that even with good inhaler technique, it is hard to inhale all of the medication and using a spacer makes this a much easier process as it removes the need to coordinate inhalation and activation

1. Check the expiry date of the inhaler
2. Ask the patient to stand up or sit up straight and lift his chin
3. Shake the inhaler well
4. Take the cap off the inhaler
5. Ask the patient to assemble the spacer and attach the inhaler to it (Fig 7.8)
6. Ask the patient to exhale completely
7. Ask the patient to place his lips firmly around the mouthpiece (Fig 7.9)
8. Ask the patient to press the canister to release a dose into the spacer
9. Ask the patient to take five slow, deep breaths
10. If more than one puff is required, wait 30 seconds before repeating the process

Make sure you inform patients about cleaning the spacer. It needs to be washed once a week in warm soapy water and left to air dry. Also, spacers need to be replaced every three to six months

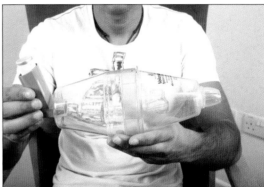
Fig 7.8: Assemble the equipment correctly

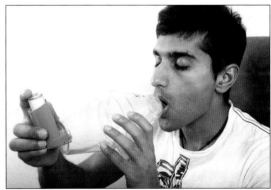
Fig 7.9: Ensure a tight seal

There are different types of spacers. For example:
- Babyhaler: in <2 year-olds (with face mask) - does not have to be upright; listen for five clicks
- Volumatic: in >2 year-olds (with or without face mask) - should be seated upright
- Aerochamber with 3 different sized masks for infants, children and adults (now the most commonly prescribed spacer in the UK)

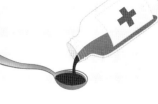

Mark Scheme for Examiner

Introduction and General Advice

Introduces self (clean hands)

Identifies patient (3 points of ID)

Ensures that consent has been obtained

Asks what the patient already knows and if they are on treatment already, ask them to demonstrate technique

Provides simple explanation of how a reliever inhaler works

Inhaler Technique

Checks expiry date

Removes cap and shakes inhaler

Sits upright or stands

Exhales

Seals lips around the mouthpiece

Inhales deeply and presses the canister to release the drug during inhalation

Removes the inhaler and holds breath for 10 seconds then breathes out slowly

Checks patient understanding

Asks the patient to demonstrate/repeat

Using a Spacer

Explains what a spacer device is and why it is used

Shakes the inhaler and attaches it to the aerochamber

Exhales completely. Seals lips around mouth piece. Presses canister once

Inhales slowly and deeply, repeat up to 4-5 times

Provides cleaning advice – rinse and air dry

Asks the patient to demonstrate/repeat

Asks the patient if they have any questions

Finishing the Consultation

Arranges a follow up appointment if necessary or offers contact details

Thanks the patient and close the consultation

General Points

Checks patient understanding throughout the consultation, avoiding medical jargon, and offers information leaflets

Maintains good eye contact; remains polite and engaged with the patient

Questions and Answers for Candidate

What are the side effects of inhaled steroids?

* Candida infection of the mouth
* Hoarseness

Rarely:
* Skin – easy bruising and thinning
* Weakened immunity – instruct patients that they should inform their doctors if ill

What are some important questions to ask a patient with chronic asthma?

* What are you like at your worst and how is your asthma normally?
* Have you ever been admitted to hospital with your asthma? What treatment did you receive?
* Have you ever been admitted to intensive care to help with your breathing?
* Do you use home oxygen, inhalers or nebulisers? Are you on any other medications for asthma?
* How many courses of steroids have you taken in the last year?
* Are there any specific triggers to your asthma?
* Have you had any chest infections in the last year?
* Can you demonstrate your inhaler technique?

Name two different types on inhaler available

* Metered dose inhalers
* Breath activated inhalers – Autohaler, Easibreathe
* Dry powder inhalers – Accuhaler

Additional Questions to Consider

1. What is the difference between moderate, severe and life-threatening asthma?
2. What is the difference between type one and type two respiratory failure?
3. What are the differentials for a presentation of acute breathlessness in a five year old child?
4. Give some examples of possible triggers for an asthma exacerbation

Station 3: PREPARING BABY FORMULA MILK

Mrs Fenton is a 29-year-old with a two-month-old child. She has decided to stop breastfeeding and wants to use baby formula milk. Please demonstrate to her how to correctly prepare baby formula milk.

Objectives

* Preparing baby formula milk

Explaining Preparing Baby Formula Milk

* Preparing milk in a sterilised manner is vital. Although rare, bacterial infections in infants can be life-threatening
* The main method used to reduce the risk of bacterial infection is to prepare each feed with boiling water, as this kills any potentially harmful bacteria
* It's critical to remember to cool the water fully before giving the feed to the infant

Preparation

* Ensure you wash your hands with soap and water before handling any of the equipment needed
* All equipment must be sterilised before each use
* Clean the work surface before you prepare the formula milk

Preparing Baby Formula Milk

1. Fill a kettle with fresh cold tap water
2. Boil the kettle
3. Leave to cool for 15-30 minutes (ensuring the temperature of the water is above 70°C)
4. Wash your hands with soap and water
5. Take out the baby's bottle, teat and cap from the steriliser (Fig 7.10)
6. Stand the baby bottle on the cleaned work surface
7. Follow the manufacturer's instructions for the formula using the specified amount of formula powder and hot water. Place the water into the bottle first, followed by the powder
8. Put the teat onto the bottle, holding the edge
9. Screw the teat onto the bottle
10. Place the cap over the teat
11. Shake the bottle firmly until the powder has dissolved
12. Allow the formula to cool quickly by running the bottle under a cold tap
13. Test the temperature of the formula using the inside of your wrist. The formula should be at body temperature so should feel tepid to the touch, not hot
14. The formula is now ready to use (Fig 7.11)

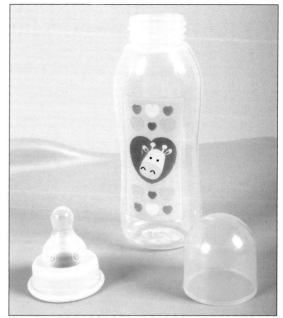

Fig 7.10: Bottle, teat, and cap

Only prepare feeds at the time they are required. Despite being prepared correctly, formula kept in the fridge is still at risk of becoming infected with bacteria. If absolutely necessary, formula can be kept in the fridge for up to 24 hours but this is not recommended. Any left-over formula should be thrown away or used within two hours

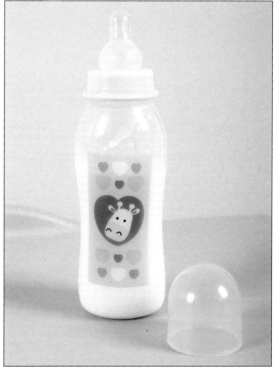

Fig 7.11: Ensure all the powder is dissolved before use

'Always ensure that you use the scoop that is provided with the formula powder to measure the correct amount of powder. If the formula is too concentrated dehydration can ensue, whilst if the formula is too weak it can eventually lead to failure to thrive'

Mark Scheme for Examiner

Introduction and General Preparation
Introduces self (clean hands)

Identifies patient (3 points of ID)

Explains procedure, identifies concerns

Cleans the work surface

Preparing Baby Formula Milk
Boils tap water

Leaves to cool

Washes hands with soap and water

Removes equipment from steriliser

Follows manufacturer's instructions for quantities of water and powder

Screws teat in place

Places on cap

Shakes firmly

Cools bottle under cold tap water and then tests temperature

Finishing
Ensures workspace is cleaned

Discusses questions with parent

Questions and Answers for Candidate

Why is it not advisable to give cow's milk to an infant under the age of 1?

Cow's milk has low levels of some nutrients, specifically iron, vitamin C and vitamin E. Cow's milk can also be a source of bacterial infection as it is not sterile

How long can prepared baby formula milk be kept unrefrigerated?

Two hours, thereafter, the formula milk should be discarded

Additional Questions to Consider

1. What are the advantages to breastfeeding?
2. How do the nutrients in baby formula compare to breast milk?
3. When might you recommend formula milk for a baby?
4. When would you consider weaning a child onto solid food?

PAEDIATRICS

8 GENERAL SKILLS

GENERAL SKILLS

Station 1: HAND WASHING

Mrs Vigus requires an abdominal examination. Please demonstrate your hand washing technique.

Objectives

- To revise the correct method of hand washing
- To understand when the use of soap and water or alcohol gel for hand washing is indicated

General Advice

Each trust will have guidelines adapted from the World Health Organisation guidelines on the 'Five Moments of Hand Hygiene'. Ensure that you are familiar with these

Hand Washing Procedure

1. Thoroughly wet hands with warm water
2. Apply liquid soap or disinfectant from dispenser
3. Wash hands using the Ayliffe technique (described below):
    - Palm to palm (Fig 8.1)
    - Palm to palm with fingers interlaced (Fig 8.2)
    - Back of left hand fingers against right hand opposing palms with fingers interlocked, then vice versa (Fig 8.3)
    - Left thumb clasped in right palm and vice versa (Fig 8.4)
    - Fingers of right hand clasped in left palm and vice versa (Fig 8.5)
4. Rinse hands thoroughly
5. Turn taps off with elbows
6. Dry hands with paper towel
7. Dispose of paper towel in clinical waste bin

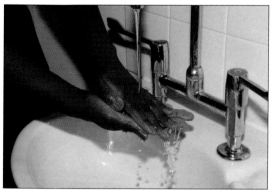

Fig 8.1: Palm to palm

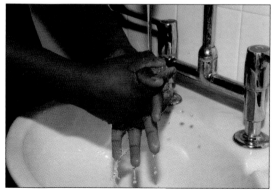

Fig 8.2: Palm to palm with fingers interlaced

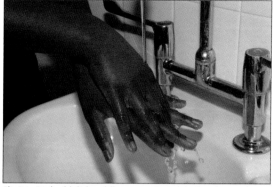

Fig 8.3: Back of left hand fingers against right hand opposing palm with fingers interlocked

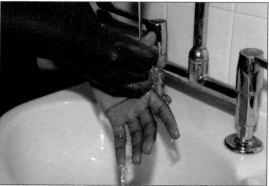

Fig 8.4: Left thumb clasped in left palm

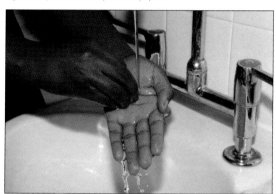

Fig 8.5: Fingers of right hand clasped in left palm

Hands should be washed with soap and water if they are visibly soiled or you have undertaken any procedure that you have used gloves for. Alcohol gel is adequate if hands are not soiled (for example entering or leaving a hospital ward). Usage of soap and water is also preferable if there is a concern about certain infections e.g. *Clostridum Difficile*

'Areas such as the thumbs and tips of the fingers are commonly missed during hand washing. Ensure that you focus on such areas'

8 // General Skills

Mark Scheme for Examiner

Hand Washing Procedure: Preparation

Wets hands with warm water   ☐ ☐ ☐ ☐ ☐

Applies soap or disinfectant   ☐ ☐ ☐ ☐ ☐

Hand Washing Procedure: Ayliffe Technique

Palm to palm   ☐ ☐ ☐ ☐ ☐

Fingers interlaced   ☐ ☐ ☐ ☐ ☐

Palm over back of hand   ☐ ☐ ☐ ☐ ☐

Thumb   ☐ ☐ ☐ ☐ ☐

Fingers   ☐ ☐ ☐ ☐ ☐

Repeats each action for both hands   ☐ ☐ ☐ ☐ ☐

Hand Washing Procedure: Finishing

Rinses hands   ☐ ☐ ☐ ☐ ☐

Turns off taps with elbows   ☐ ☐ ☐ ☐ ☐

Dries hands with paper towel   ☐ ☐ ☐ ☐ ☐

Disposes of paper towel   ☐ ☐ ☐ ☐ ☐

Questions and Answers for Candidate

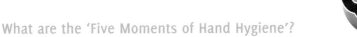

Additional Questions to Consider

What are the 'Five Moments of Hand Hygiene'?

1. Prior to patient contact
2. Before an aseptic task
3. After exposure to bodily fluid
4. After patient contact
5. After contact with patient surroundings

Who must perform hand hygiene?

- Healthcare professionals
- Patients
- Visitors
- Allied health professionals

Can gloves be a substitute for hand washing?

- No, if gloves are to be worn, hands must be washed before they are put on and after they are removed

1. How can healthcare-related infections be transmitted?
2. What would you do if you saw a colleague with poor hand washing skills?
3. How might you prevent hand washing related dermatitis?

Mrs Tower is a 69-year-old woman who is being cared for on the high dependency unit. She has been isolated following positive swabs for MRSA, has a long-term urinary catheter, a central venous catheter and is being fed by a NG tube. Please discuss with the examiner the infection control issues surrounding this patient.

Objectives

- To understand the use of personal protective equipment
- To understand the infection control aspects of urinary catheters
- To understand the infection control aspects of enteral feeding
- To understand the infection control aspects of central venous catheters

General Advice

Each trust will have guidelines for infection control adapted from NICE guidelines. Ensure that you are familiar with your Trust's policies. Handwashing is discussed in the previous station

Personal Protective Equipment

What can you tell me about personal protective equipment (PPE)?

1. 'PPE protects infection passing between me and my patient'
2. 'I have seen gloves, aprons, goggles and face masks commonly used. Gloves are indicated if I am to have any contact with wounds, bodily fluids or blood. Aprons are indicated if there is a risk of bodily fluids splashing onto my clothes. Goggles and face masks are indicated if there is a risk of bodily fluids splashing into my face or eyes'
3. 'In many Trusts, patients who are isolated in a side room for infection control purposes also require healthcare professionals to wear an apron and gloves before entering the room'
4. 'I am aware of other equipment such as respirators which are used for airborne infections'

Aprons, gloves and face masks are single use only
After disposing of the items in a clinical waste bin it is important to wash your hands

Long-term Urinary Catheters

What are the important infection control aspects to consider with regards to urinary catheters?

1. 'Long-term catheters are only used once other methods of management have been considered or tried'
2. 'Catheters should be inserted using an aseptic technique and changed as per manufactures recommendations'
3. 'Patients with long-term catheters should be educated on managing their catheter using basic infection control principles'
4. 'Patients with a history of recurrent urinary tract infections or cardiac defects should have antibiotic cover when changing catheters'

Enteral Feeding

What are the important infection control aspects to consider with regards to enteral feeding?

1. 'Enteral feeds should be, where possible, ready-to-use. Feeds that require diluting or reconstituting are at higher risk of contamination'
2. 'Enteral feeding tubes should be flushed regularly before and after each use with cooled boiled water or sterile water according to Trust protocol'
3. 'When connecting the feed with the administration system, there should be minimal handling to reduce the infection risk'

Central Venous Catheters

What are the important infection control aspects to consider with regards to central venous catheters?

1. 'Central venous catheters must be handled using an aseptic technique, preferably with sterile gloves'
2. 'Dressings over the insertion site should be transparent to allow the site to be assessed for signs of infection, such as: erythema, discharge and warmth. Dressings should be changed at least once a week'
3. 'Catheter infection ports are at high risk for infection so should be cleaned using an alcohol wipe before and after each use'
4. 'Catheter ports should be clearly labelled in accordance with their use. The label is placed at the distal end of the infusion line. The use of each port should be clearly documented in the patient's notes. Examples of possible labels include: blood sampling; medication administration or blood administration'

Mark Scheme for Examiner

Personal Protective Equipment

Discusses indications ☐ ☐ ☐ ☐ ☐

Discusses common personal protective equipment e.g. gloves ☐ ☐ ☐ ☐ ☐

Discusses less common personal protective equipment e.g. respirators ☐ ☐ ☐ ☐ ☐

Long-term Urinary Catheters

Discusses catheter insertion ☐ ☐ ☐ ☐ ☐

Discusses antibiotic use ☐ ☐ ☐ ☐ ☐

Discusses basic infection control procedures for long term catheters ☐ ☐ ☐ ☐ ☐

Enteral Feeding

Discusses different feeds e.g. ready to use vs those requiring preparation ☐ ☐ ☐ ☐ ☐

Discusses process of giving feeds ☐ ☐ ☐ ☐ ☐

Central Venous Catheter

Discusses handing central venous catheters ☐ ☐ ☐ ☐ ☐

Discusses monitoring of insertion site ☐ ☐ ☐ ☐ ☐

Discusses labelling catheters ☐ ☐ ☐ ☐ ☐

Questions and Answers for Candidate

When should wearing a respirator (protective mask) be considered?

- Anyone coming in contact with a patient with a communicable disease spread through the air, e.g. possible Avian flu

Additional Questions to Consider

1. What pathogens might cause a urinary tract infection?
2. Which commensals normally colonise on our skin?
3. What are the complications of having a "long-line" inserted?
4. What are the complications of enteral feeding?

Station 3: MANUAL HANDLING

Mr Counter is an 89-year-old man admitted three weeks ago following a stroke. He has reduced power in his left arm and leg and finds it hard to mobilise on the ward. Please discuss how you would assess this patient for a task involving manual handling, and describe some of the common manual handling techniques used on the ward.

Objectives

- To assess a manual handling task for a patient
- To understand independent movement methods
- To understand basic assisted techniques for adults

General Advice

Each trust will have guidelines for manual handling and have regular update courses which you should attend. Where possible, patients should be encouraged to mobilise by themselves. If manual handling is required, a full assessment must be made prior to each task

Manual Handling Assessment

How would you assess a patient manual handling task?

1. 'I would need to consider the patient, the nature of the task, the environment and the equipment available'
2. 'When assessing the patient, I need to consider factors including their ability, understanding, weight, height and co-operation'
3. 'When assessing the nature of the task, I need to consider what the task involves, the separate stages of the task and how I will carry out the task'
4. 'When assessing the environment, I need to determine whether it is suitable and safe to undertake the manual handling task, considering lighting, hazards and accessibility'
5. 'When assessing the equipment available, I need to ensure I am aware of the equipment within my department, whether it is suitable and safe to use and that the user is trained to use it'

Different departments will store different types of manual handling equipment. Common equipment includes:
- Hand blocks
- Slide sheets
- Bed pulls
- Patslide
- Hoists

Independent Movement Methods

Discuss independent movement methods...

1. 'These methods provide minimal support to patients, allowing them to remain mobile and independent. These methods should only be utilised if they are deemed safe for your patient'
2. 'These methods involve talking patients through methods to assist with mobilising. Examples of these methods include:

Sitting up from lying (Fig 8.6) Tell the patient to:
1. Bend your knees
2. Roll towards your strong arm
3. Push up with both arms to sitting

Each patient who has problems with mobility and needs assistance should have an up-to-date manual handling assessment, usually located in the nursing notes

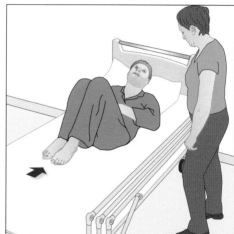

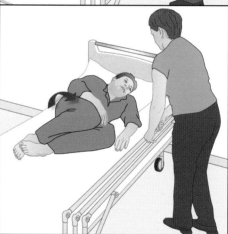

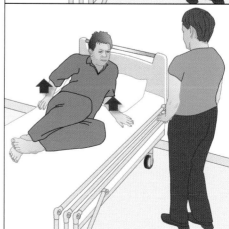

Fig 8.6: 3 steps used to sit from lying

Shuffling back up the bed (Fig 8.7) **Tell the patient to:**
1. Sit upright
2. Lean forwards
3. Place both hands behind your hips
4. Bend both knees
5. Push down with your hands and lift buttocks
6. Push up the bed using heels, not letting your buttocks drag on the sheets

Standing from sitting (Fig 8.8) **Tell the patient to:**
1. Shuffle buttocks to the front of the chair
2. Place both feet flat on the floor under your knees
3. Grip the armrest with both hands
4. Lean forwards over your knees
5. Push upwards using your hands and legs to stand'

Assisted Techniques

Discuss assisted techniques...

1. 'Assisted techniques are in place to ensure that patients are moved in a safe and careful manner'
2. 'Where possible independent movement methods are tried before an assisted technique is used'
3. 'An assisted technique should only be undertaken following a full manual handling assessment and if the appropriate number of staff to perform the task are available'
4. 'Examples of such techniques include:
   - Turning a patient in bed using a slide sheet
   - Assisting a patient to sit from lying
   - Sliding a patient up the bed using a slide sheet
   - Transferring a patient between beds
   - Assisting a patient to stand from sitting in a chair'

Reference
http://www.hse.gov.uk/pubns/indg143.pdf

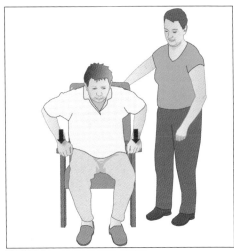

Fig 8.7: How to direct a patient to shuffle up the bed

Fig 8.8: How to stand from sitting

Mark Scheme for Examiner

Manual Handling Assessment

Assesses patient – ability, understanding, height, weight, co-operation

☐ ☐ ☐ ☐ ☐

Assesses task

☐ ☐ ☐ ☐ ☐

Assesses environment

☐ ☐ ☐ ☐ ☐

Assesses equipment

☐ ☐ ☐ ☐ ☐

Independent Moving Methods

Discusses what these methods are

☐ ☐ ☐ ☐ ☐

Discusses some examples

☐ ☐ ☐ ☐ ☐

Discusses which patients they would be indicated in

☐ ☐ ☐ ☐ ☐

Assisted Techniques

Discusses what these methods are

☐ ☐ ☐ ☐ ☐

Discusses some examples

☐ ☐ ☐ ☐ ☐

Discusses which patients they would be indicated in

☐ ☐ ☐ ☐ ☐

GENERAL SKILLS

Questions and Answers for Candidate

Why does a manual handling assessment have to be undertaken?

- To ensure patient safety
- To ensure staff safety
- To ensure the patient is moved in the best possible way, encouraging independence where possible

Once an assessment has been carried out for a task, does it have to be repeated?

- Only if the patient's ability, understanding or co-operation changes

Additional Questions to Consider

1. What assessment tools could you utilise to assess a patient's understanding?
2. How would you calculate a patient's BMI?
3. Who should be trained in manual handling techniques?

Station 4: DEATH CERTIFICATION

You are asked to verify a death and to write a death certificate. Your patient is Mrs Alice Jayne Morgue DOB: 14.02.1945. She had known angina and passed away today (26.12.2013) in hospital at 15:52. She was admitted 3 days ago with a STEMI after collapsing in the street whilst shopping. She was being treated for type II diabetes (diagnosed in 1995) and hypertension (diagnosed in 2000). She was not for resuscitation and was found dead in her bed during the night.

Objectives

- Learn how to verify a death
- Learn how to write a death certificate
- Learn how to complete a cremation form

Examine the patient to determine the following:

- No response to a painful stimuli (sternal rub or supraorbital pressure)
- Absence of carotid pulse for over one minute
- Absence of breath sounds for over one minute
- Absence of heart sounds for over one minute
- Pupils dilated and unresponsive to light

Always remember to:

- Record the date and time of death in the notes. The time of death is taken when the death is verified and not before
- Leave the patient (mannequin) in a dignified manner and cover the body with a sheet up to the neck

Writing a Death Certificate

- Make sure you understand and know the case. You do not have to have been present at the death or have been the doctor that verified it but you must have seen the patient within the last two weeks prior to death
- Ask about the specific hospital protocol for death certificates. Some hospitals expect you, as a junior doctor, to discuss the death with a consultant before issuing the certificate
- Write in block capitals and in black ink
- Avoid medical abbreviations
- Write the patient's full name
- When writing the date of death, put the date in words
- State the place of death
- Remember to check the patient's employment history, as some industrial diseases attract financial compensation (e.g. exposure to asbestos)

You **must** circle either:

1. The certified cause of death takes account of information obtained from post-mortem
2. Information from post-mortem may be available later
3. Post-mortem not being held

You must circle either:

a) Seen after death by me
b) Seen after death by another medical practitioner but not by me
c) Not seen by a medical practitioner

'The relatives may wish to remain while you verify the death of the patient. If this is the case, make sure you explain what you are going to do as otherwise they may be distressed when you are assessing for a response to a painful stimuli'

Cause of Death

- Write the cause (e.g. myocardial infarction) rather than mode of death (coma, syncope, and cardiac arrest are modes of death)
- If you do not know the cause of death, you may not be able to issue the death certificate

State whether the case has been reported to the coroner (or Procurator Fiscal in Scotland)

Part I

- State the disease or condition directly leading to death on the first line, Part I (a)
- Complete the sequence of conditions leading to death on subsequent lines

For example, Part 1a: Intrapulmonary haemorrhage, Part 1b: Squamous cell carcinoma of the lung

Part II

- State significant conditions or diseases that contributed to the death, but which are not part of any sequence leading directly to death. For example, diabetes mellitus
- Duration of all conditions listed in Part 1 and Part 2 should be listed
- Print your name clearly after your signature and add your medical qualification as registered with the GMC. If obtained in another country, state which university town it was obtained in and the year it was awarded
- Give the name of the Consultant responsible for the care of the patient

Copy what has been written on the death certificate into the medical notes, and in the death certificate booklet on the stub in the spaces provided. It is often useful to note which family members were present at the time of death, and whether the GP has been informed yet

Cremation Forms

- Do not complete the cremation form until you know that the case is not being investigated by the Coroner or Procurator Fiscal and a death certificate has been issued
- The patient must have been seen by the certifying doctor in the last two weeks of life
- The first part can be filled in by any doctor, but they MUST have seen the patient alive within the last two weeks of life and then seen and examined the body after death
- The presence of pacemakers or any type of radioactive implant must be recorded as these may preclude cremation unless they are removed
- All parts of the form must be completed in full and then signed
- After filling out the first part of the form, a second doctor (who has been fully registered for more than five years) must fill out the second part
- The form should not be given to the relatives but will be passed to the undertakers, usually via the mortuary staff or bereavement officers

'As a junior doctor you may be the one who fills out death certificates and cremation forms. It is important that you make sure you don't rush these forms and you discuss the cause of death with the team to confirm that the details you write down are correct. If in any doubt regarding what to put on the form, then the local coroner's officers are a good resource and may be able to help'

Please complete the death certificate for Mrs Morgue

Medical certificate of cause of death

Name of deceased

Date of death	Day	Month	Year	Time of death	Hour	Min

Place of death

Cause of death

I hereby certify that to the best of my knowledge and belief, the cause of death was as stated below:

1. Disease or condition directly leading to death

Antecedent causes

Morbid conditions, if any, giving rise to above cause, stating the underlying condition last

a.)

b.)

c.)

d.)

Approximate interval between onset and death

Years	Months	Days

2. Other significant conditions contributing to the death, but not related to the disease or condition causing it

---

Please tick the relevant box

Post mortem

PM1 ☐ Post mortem has been done and information is included above

PM2 ☐ Post mortem information may be available later

PM3 ☐ No post mortem is being done

Procurator fiscal/coroner

PF ☐ This death has been reported to the procurator fiscal/coroner

Extra information for statistical purposes

X ☐ I may later be able to supply the Registrar General with additional information

Attendance on deceased

A1 ☐ I was in attendance upon the deceased during last illness

A2 ☐ I was not in attendance upon the deceased during last illness: the doctor who was is unable to provide the certificate

A3 ☐ No doctor was in attendance on the deceased

Signature

Name in BLOCK CAPITALS

Official address

Date:

For a death in hospital

Name of the consultant responsible

Counterfoil – Medical certificate of cause of death

Name of deceased

Date of death

Place of death

Please circle as appropriate

Post mortem	PM1 or	PM2 or	PM3	
Procurator fiscal/coroner	PF			
Extra information	X			
Attendance on decreased	A1	A2	A3	

Cause of death

I (a)

(b)

(c)

(d)

II

Date of certificate

Mark Scheme for Examiner

Introduction and General Preparation

Introduces self to relatives, if present (cleans hands)
☐ ☐ ☐ ☐ ☐

Explains the process to family members
☐ ☐ ☐ ☐ ☐

Verification of death

Assesses for a painful stimulus
☐ ☐ ☐ ☐ ☐

Palpates for a carotid pulse for one minute
☐ ☐ ☐ ☐ ☐

Auscultates for heart sounds and breath sounds for a minute each
☐ ☐ ☐ ☐ ☐

Assesses pupil size and response
☐ ☐ ☐ ☐ ☐

Documents the death in the notes correctly
☐ ☐ ☐ ☐ ☐

Leaves the patient in an appropriate state
☐ ☐ ☐ ☐ ☐

Writing a death certificate

Writes in black ink, block capitals, without abbreviations
☐ ☐ ☐ ☐ ☐

Fills in the patient details, place, date and time of death correctly
☐ ☐ ☐ ☐ ☐

Chooses appropriate option about post-mortem, reporting to procurator fiscal/coroner and if the doctor filling out the certificate was present at time of death
☐ ☐ ☐ ☐ ☐

Fills in cause of death appropriately
☐ ☐ ☐ ☐ ☐

Fills in co-morbidities appropriately
☐ ☐ ☐ ☐ ☐

Fills in personal details and consultant details
☐ ☐ ☐ ☐ ☐

Signs the document
☐ ☐ ☐ ☐ ☐

Questions and Answers for Candidate

Give some examples of when a death might be reported to a coroner (or procurator fiscal)

- Any uncertified death (i.e. for which the clinician is unable or unwilling to issue a death certificate)
- Any death that is sudden and unexpected, or that is due to any violent, suspicious or unexplained cause
- Any death for which the cause is known but the patient has not been seen within the last two weeks of life
- Any death resulting from an accident at work or arising out of the use of a vehicle, or involving burns or scalds, or a fire or an explosion, or of any other similar cause. This includes deaths occurring as a late result of trauma (i.e. months afterwards)
- Any death due to poisoning, including drug overdose (even as a late result)
- Any death resulting from an industrial disease
- Any death in hospital occurring within 24 hours of admission
- Any death where circumstances indicate that suicide is a possibility
- Any death where there are indications that it occurred as a result of medical mishap
- Any death following an abortion or attempted abortion
- Any death where the circumstances seem to indicate fault or neglect on the part of another person or organisation including hospitals
- Any death occurring as a result of food poisoning or a notifiable infectious disease
- Any death of a foster child

Additional Questions to Consider

1. Who is the death certificate given to?
2. What is the difference between decorticate and decerebrate movements?
3. Who can issue a death certificate?